AF730855

MISS COTTON'S

BIG HERB BOOK

— herbal recipes and remedies —

This Belongs in Every Home!

Yolanda *Miss Cotton* Justice

Master Herbalist

Published in USA by Trinity Publishing Company

Book Cover & Formatting: Paul Nomshan of Trinity Publishing Company

Paperback ISBN: 978-1-964707-68-6
eBook ISBN: 978-1-964707-69-3

Dedication

This book is dedicated to all of my ancestors who have gone on before me, praying that someone keeps the tradition of natural medicine going.

I am also dedicating this book to my two sons, Marcos and Ledarion, and my grandchildren, Vivian, Aiden, Austin, Jacob, Brandon, Alyssa, Adonis, Andrew, Naomi, and the future generations to come. I pray that this book is sitting on the shelf of their homes one day.

Disclaimer:

I am not a doctor, and I do not make medical claims. As an herbalist, I share knowledge based on traditional and personal experiences.

-Always consult with a qualified healthcare professional before using any herbal remedies or making changes to your health regimen.

Contents

Preface

If you are reading this book, you have made a huge step in naturally taking care of this vessel called our bodies. Congratulations to you. You most likely want to feel empowered to care for your own self and your family with the natural herbs instead of using over-the-counter or prescription pharmaceuticals for ailments that are coming. You may be seeking some knowledge about the traditional ways of healing a health issue that has been ongoing. Perhaps you have already started to explore herbal medicine, and you have developed a serious interest in it, and you are ready to learn how to incorporate herbal medicines into your daily self-care routine. Whatever your reason, I thank you, and I invite you to explore the recipes that are in this book at your own pace and use them as needed.

My name is Yolanda Justice, and I have been raised in herbalism my whole life. My grandmother, Naomi Ruth Bennett Ransom, was Native American and African. She leaned heavily on her Native American roots when it came to natural medicine. She had a garden in her backyard with a variety of herbs that she pulled from for all medical emergencies in our home. We rarely visited the hospital. She always had her own remedies for ailments that others would seek hospital treatment for.

One incident that sticks out in my mind vividly is when I was a very little girl jumping off the car with my little brother. We were about five and six. I jumped off the car successfully, but when it was my little brother's turn, he landed on a stick, and it went straight through his leg around the thigh area. He raised himself off of the ground and ran into the house crying hysterically.

I was trailing behind fearfully because I was the one who talked him into jumping off of the car. My grandmother came into the living room and told my brother to calm down. Her voice was so low and steady that it confused us. There was blood shooting everywhere out of my brother's leg, and for us, she was too calm. She folded a big towel and placed it on the sofa. She instructed my brother to lay his leg on top of the towel. By this time, I could see that the stick had left a quarter-sized hole piercing through his leg.

My grandmother broke a large piece of aloe from her plant and squeezed the gel into the hole of my brother's leg. At this point as a child, I am thinking that my grandmother has lost her mind. Why wasn't anyone rushing my brother to the hospital like they did on TV when people were bleeding like that?

As I watched her continue to squeeze the aloe vera gel into my brother's leg, I noticed something remarkable. The blood stopped shooting out of his leg, and it started congealing into a thick gel. The aloe vera actually stopped the bleeding on my brother's leg long enough for her to finish cleaning it off and wrapping both sides of his leg up with an unknown substance. That was the day I was amazed by how my grandmother handled the situation, and it was also when I learned about the healing power of aloe vera. It not only healed and soothed our little burns that we got frequently; it also helped blood to congeal quickly.

My brother's leg eventually healed, and there was a shiny quarter-size scar left for proof. In hindsight, he probably should have gotten stitches and had his leg checked for any tendon damage, but back then we were just happy that the bleeding stopped. My brother still has the scar on his leg, and it healed just fine.

My grandmother was the person that everyone came to for herbal remedies or just to be touched by her healing hands until the day she transitioned from this Earth in 2005. This book is the accumulation of things that my grandmother taught me and also things that I learned in my studies to acquire my Master Herbalist Certification. During my studies to become a master herbalist, I was often juggling several books to get information about one herb. My motivation for creating this book is for you to have an inclusive, concise reference that is easy for you to use.

The first chapter will give you a list of common herbs that are used with the most useful delivery methods and applications along with information about which one is best suited to what type of sickness or ailment and why. My goal is to equip you with natural remedies that you can use in your home. I understand that some things still need medical attention, but there are so many herbs that were created to deal with our health issues naturally.

More and more I am seeing people return to the old ways of relying on our self-knowledge and traditional medicine. Herbal medicine is a very important tool that helps us live healthier lives and actively participate and improve our overall health naturally. You may already use herbs as part of your daily regimen or step it up a bit when you see something acute showing up.

The study of the herbs and plants and their uses and what makes them powerful healing agents gives you the framework for creating treatments. This book will address some of the most common complaints that people deal with. I am not a medical doctor; I am someone who is well versed in the use of natural herbs. My advice is to use your own discretion and be careful about combining substances that could be toxic to your body. Always research the herbs you are using and their counter actions to make sure you are using them safely and properly.

1

Healing Herbs and Their Uses

ALFALFA—Medicago sativa

Parts used: Aerial parts
Taste/Smell: Bland
Tendencies: Cooling, moisturizing

Uses:

- Anti-inflammatory, Nutritive, Diuretic, Phytoestrogen.
- Alfalfa contains a very high vitamin and mineral content; it is rich in carotene, calcium, protein, trace minerals, and vitamins K and E. It also has water-soluble vitamins. Alfalfa has been known to stimulate and increase lactation and the quality of breast milk. Some people have used it as a tonic in several chronic degenerative diseases. Alfalfa has also been shown to decrease the level of cholesterol. Alfalfa is not recommended for someone dealing with lupus because it may cause stimulation of the immune system by L-canavanine.

ALOE VERA—Aloe barbadensis

Parts Used: The whole leaf
Taste/Smell: The outer leaf has a bitter taste, but the mucilage on the inside has a pleasant taste.
Tendencies: Cooling, drying, stimulating.

Uses:

- Laxative, increases menstrual flow, stimulates the flow of bile from the liver, promotes the appetite, and assists with digestion.
- Aloe Vera has natural cooling, soothing, and moisturizing properties. It is often used to treat burns. It is very helpful with wound healing and pain relief, and it is also inexpensive.
- Aloe Vera also improves your digestive health. When it is consumed, it helps to soothe your digestive tract and cure stomach ailments, including irritable bowel syndrome (IBS).
- Aloe Vera is used in toothpaste and mouthwash as a natural option to improve oral hygiene and reduce plaque. Another great thing about aloe is its ability to help clear up acne.

ANISE—Pimpinella Ansium

Parts Used: Ripe seeds
Taste/Smell: Sweet and aromatic
Tendencies: Warming

Uses:

- Relieves flatulence, flavoring agent, expectorant, mild anti-spasmodic, lactation inducer.
- Anise is commonly used for children's complaints due to its great taste and its actions. It is used for coughs, asthma, bronchitis, and as a digestive aid. Anise is also used to increase overall secretions such as urine, sweating, milk flow, and menstruation. It is not recommended to use it while pregnant unless it is under the guidance of a trained professional.

ARNICA—Arnica spp. in the aster family

Parts Used: Fresh whole plants or the flower heads
Taste/Smell: Light and flowery

Uses:

- Stimulate circulation, anti-inflammatory, bactericidal, mild analgesic, enhance the immune system, anticoagulant, topical counter irritant.
- Arnica is used either internally or externally for musculoskeletal injuries such as strains, sprains, rheumatism, bruises, sore muscles, and varicose veins. Internally, it is used for angina and trauma calls to tissues as well as helping with mental trauma.
- Long term use in high concentrations is not recommended due to the possibility of developing skin irritations. It should be discontinued at the first sign of redness. I only trained professionals should use this herb internally. It is also not recommended for pregnant women to ingest.

ASHWAGANDHA- Withania somnifera

Parts Used: Root
Taste/Smell: Bitter, flowery and earthy.
Tendencies: Uplifting

Uses:

- Helps your body cope with stress, anxiety, and fatigue. Anti-inflammatory, adaptogenic, and lowers blood pressure.
- Ashwagandha supports strength, endurance, vitality, and rejuvenation. This herb is really helpful for people who are exhausted, debilitated, under stress, agitated, or just exhausted. Even though other parts of the plant have been used the root is the part that is usually used for herbal medicine. The root is used for stress-induced health conditions, anemia with emaciation, nervous exhaustion, impotence, chronic inflammation, and cognitive function deficits such as those with hypertension and aging.

Ashwagandha is not recommended to use during pregnancy. The unprocessed leaves should not be ingested.

ASTRAGALUS- Astragalus membranaceus

Parts Used: Root
Taste/Smell: Moistening, sweet
Tendencies: Slightly warming, circulates moisture.

Uses:

- Activates or suppresses immune function, adaptogenic, anti-tumor activity, antioxidant, protects kidney function, protects against WBC drops during chemo, hypotensive, diuretic.
- Astragalus has been used for centuries in traditional Chinese medicine. It is known to enhance the immune system, and it reduces inflammation. It is also used to help treat heart conditions, kidney disease, and lower blood sugar levels.

BILBERRY/HUCKLEBERRY—Vaccinium spp. in the heath family

Parts Used: Leaves and berries
Taste/Smell: The berries are sweet and tart, and the leaves are astringent.

Uses:

- Hypoglycemic,anti-inflammatory,neuroprotective, antioxidant, anti-mutagenic.
- Bilberry leaves have been used for diabetes, as a urinary tract antiseptic, and for diarrhea. The berries have also been used for conditions that have resulted from diabetes. It is not recommended to consume too many of the berries because of the high sugar content, but many people use them without problems and have benefited from them. The berries are used to support vision

and to help with circulatory problems, including varicose veins, hemorrhoids, and easy bruising.

BLACK COHOSH—Actaea racemosa

Parts Used: Rhizomes and roots
Taste/Smell: Sharp, spicy, bitter, acrid

Uses:

- Sedative, diaphoretic, antispasmodic, digestive stimulant, mild expectorant, hypotensive, female reproductive tract tonic, anti-inflammatory.
- Black Cohosh is often used for menstrual cramps, amenorrhea, late menstruation, endometriosis, menopausal symptoms, or post-hysterectomy. It also is used to help joint inflammation and rheumatism. It is a good herb for the first phases of influenza when there are aching muscles, acute fever, and chilliness. It is thought that the salicylic acid in black cohosh helps to alleviate myalgia and neuralgia. It also has an anti-inflammatory effect that alleviates pain. It increases and normalizes uterine **contractions during labor**; it is also good for the after pains after labor. Black Cohosh has an amazing effect on calming the central nervous system. It is well known to help with emotional irritability or depression. If your anxiety triggers physical responses like tremors, Black Cohosh is very helpful and should be taken as a formula. It is excellent for controlling symptoms of menopause and hot flashes. Black Cohosh is a smooth muscle relaxant and is often used to calm muscle tension.

BLADDERWRACK- Fucus vesiculosus

Parts Used: Fronds (thallus)
Taste/Smell: Mucilaginous, salty
Tendencies: Cooling

Uses:

- Diuretic, mucilaginous, anti-inflammatory, immunomodulator
- Bladderwrack helps to improve nutrition by supplying key minerals and Trace elements such as iodine. This is in the form of inorganic salts and iodine that are bound to proteins and lipids. It is indicated that hypothyroidism due to the lack of iodine. It is not recommended to use this herb in hypothyroidism unless it is under the guidance of a trained practitioner or if there is excessive circulating iodine. Iodine is capable of entering into breast milk and it produces an emaciating effect on infants. This is made some people feel that the seaweeds like bladder rack should be used with caution when breastfeeding and during pregnancy.

BLESSED THISTLE—Cnicus benedictus

Parts Used: Aerial parts in flower
Taste/Smell: Aromatic and bitter
Tendencies: Cooling

Uses:

- Appetite enhancer
- Blessed thistle is used to stimulate an appetite and help with digestion. It promotes the secretion of gastric juices and saliva. It has been used as a bitter tonic to help with gastrointestinal colic with gas and loose stools, gallbladder issues, and anorexia. It may also be used to stimulate lactation. It is not recommended to use in high doses because it may irritate the stomach lining and cause vomiting. Do not use during pregnancy.

BURDOCK ROOT—Arctium lappa

Parts Used: Roots

Taste/Smell: It is initially sweet, after which it has bitter tones, slightly mucilaginous

Uses:

- Antibacterial, anti-inflammatory, antifungal, diuretic, digestive stimulant, liver tonic, anti-mutagenic, promotes blood and lymph circulation, mild laxative.
- Burdock root, traditionally known as a liver herb, offers consistent support in detoxing your body and its processes. This burdock root offers consistent support that detoxifies your body and aids in the healing process of the stomach lining. The root is most commonly used, but the leaves are also utilized. When the leaves are used, they promote mild bile stimulation and are used as a wash for poison oak or poison ivy. Burdock root is beneficial for those in need of more grounding in their lives. It is also used for chronic skin eruptions such as eczema, boils, acne psoriasis, styes, and carbuncles. It is beneficial for sciatica, gout, and arthritis. Burdock road is also commonly used to normalize the female menstrual cycle, during menopause and for mastitis.
- If you find yourself overwhelmed with scattered thoughts or responsibilities, or if your mind is often elsewhere, this herb is excellent for you. If you have a constant high energy level or tend to be daydreaming, burdock root is highly suitable. However, exercise caution if you already exhibit signs of a depressive nature.

CALENDULA—Calendula *officinalis* in the Asteraceae or Aster family

Part used: Flowers prior to fully opening
Taste/smell: Slightly bitter, salty
Tendencies: Drying

Uses:

- Antiseptic, Anti-inflammatory, Lymphagogue, Choleretic, Demulcent.
- Calendula is an herb known for its ability to bring tissues together to expedite natural healing. Naturally antibacterial, it is a great herb for keeping areas free from infection while promoting wound healing. Calendula is commonly used internally for conditions such as gastritis, menstrual pain, fever, and occasional recurring vomiting.

CATNIP—Nepeta cataria in the Lamiaceae or Mint family

Part used: Aerial parts
Taste/smell: Bitter
Tendencies: Cooling and drying

Uses:

- Relaxing diaphoretic, antispasmodic, carminative, nervine, mild sedative.
- Due to catnip being suitable for infants and children, it is used in childhood fevers and colic. It is also used to produce perspiration and lower fevers, help with restlessness, nervous irritation, nervous headaches, and insomnia. Not recommended to use during pregnancy.

CELERY—Apium graveolens

Parts Used: Seeds
Taste/Smell: Very mildly bitter

Uses:

- Emotional support
- Celery is an herb that is sometimes used for emotional support, making it a favorite go-to herb for anxiety. It can alleviate stress and help with anxiety symptoms. Many individuals who try celery seeds immediately report feeling a sense of calm that they have not experienced in a long time. Celery also helps blood flow and lowers your blood pressure.

CHAMOMILE—Matricaria *recutita* in the Asteraceae or Aster family

Parts used: Fresh flowers prior to fully opening. Fresh or dry flowers can be used.
Taste/smell: Sweet, aromatic, slightly bitter.

Uses:

- Antispasmodic, anti-inflammatory, anti-allergenic, analgesic, antipyretic, antiseptic, antibacterial, antifungal.
- Chamomile is mostly known for its use in teas to aid in sleeping. This herb also provides numerous healing benefits. Chamomile is effective in alleviating stomach issues, skin irritation, allergies, eye pain, an irregular menstrual cycle, stress, hemorrhoids, toothaches, and lower back pain. It is also beneficial for children, easing stomach discomfort and headaches. Chamomile can be consumed in teas or glycerin-based tinctures.

CHASTE TREE BERRY—Vitex agnus castus in the Verbenaceae or Verbena family

Parts used: Fruits
Taste/smell: Pungent and peppery
Tendencies: Drying

Use:

- Female reproductive tract regulator
- Chasteberry is used for PMS, endometriosis, menstrual cramps, premenstrual herpes, premenstrual acne, and menopause with hot flashes. Chaste tree has been used to treat menstrual cycle problems and pain, premenstrual syndrome, and menopause. Chaste tree berries may help stimulate progesterone. This is a female hormone that rises two weeks before menstruation. It may help normalize estrogen and progesterone.
- It is not recommended to take this during pregnancy because it stimulates contractions.

CINNAMON—Cinnamomum verum in the Lauraceae family

Parts used: Inner bark
Taste/Smell: Spicy, aromatic, sweet
Tendencies: Drying, heating, stimulating

Use:

- Astringent, diaphoretic, aromatic stimulant, carminative, hemostatic, antiseptic, flavoring, antibacterial, antifungal, gastrointestinal tonic, antioxidant.
- Cinnamon, in addition to being an antioxidant, anti-inflammatory, antidiabetic, antimicrobial, anticancer, lipid-lowering, and cardiovascular-disease-lowering compound, has also been reported to have activities against neurological disorders, such as Parkinson's and Alzheimer's diseases.

COLTSFOOT—Tussilago farfara

Parts Used: Leaves
Taste/Smell: Smooth, medicinal-like sweet

Uses:

- Immune defense, clear lungs
- ColtsFoot is a respiratory herb that targets the opening of breathing pathways to clear phlegm and lung constriction. It is a natural antimicrobial agent that soothes the respiratory tract, making it helpful for dry coughs and sore throats.

CORN SILK—Zea mays in the Poaceae family

Parts used: Fresh or dried corn silk
Taste/smell: Sweet, mucilaginous, characteristic corn smell
Tendencies: Cooling and drying

Uses:

- Soothing, toning, demulcent, diuretic, antimicrobial, antiseptic
- Corn silk is used for inflammatory states of the kidneys and bladder. It is healing to the urinary tract and helps restore normal tissue tone and function. It is specifically used to treat edema, cystitis, gout, nephritis, kidney stones, as well as prostatitis, benign prostatic hyperplasia (BPH), and similar ailments. Corn silk is safe for children with enuresis (bedwetting).

CRAMP BARK—Viburnum opulus in the Caprifoliaceae or honeysuckle family

Parts used: Bark
Taste/smell: Astringent, aromatic
Tendencies: Drying

Uses:

- Antispasmodic, astringent, nervine, hypotensive, carminative, restores balance in voluntary and involuntary muscle spasms, anti-inflammatory.
- Cramp Bark is utilized to relax and smooth muscles. It is commonly employed for uterine cramping, yet it can have effects on any smooth muscle in the body. It is a valuable addition to any reproductive blend.
- It is also known to be helpful with treating asthma and threatened miscarriage where there are spasms in the uterus. It has been used to prevent habitual abortions, morning sickness, premature contractions, and hemorrhage during labor and postpartum. As a skeletal muscle relaxant, it is wonderful for alleviating leg cramps.

DANDELION—Taraxacum officinalis in the Asteraceae or Aster family

Part Used: Whole plant, leaves, flowers, roots
Taste/Smell: Leaves and root are somewhat bitter but also slightly sweet taste in the root
Tendencies: Cooling and drying

Uses:

- Diuretic, whole plant, especially the leaf, mild laxative, choleretic, and anti-platelet aggregating action.
- Dandelion is known for helping the body clear toxins, so they are often referred to as a blood cleanser. The leaves are diuretic and help the body maintain a healthy water balance. Some people have

even said that dandelion successfully reduces rheumatism, perhaps due to its ability to clear the body of waste byproducts. Dandelion is healing and protective while also stimulating to the liver. It is indicated for many female problems and skin diseases due to its action on the liver and is specific for liver/gallbladder/digestive headaches. The whole plant, especially the root, is beneficial to the liver.

DONG QUAI—Angelica sinensis in the Umbelliferae or Parsley family

Part used: Root
Taste/smell: Sweet, bitter, slightly pungent
Tendencies: Warming, moistening, stimulating

Uses:

- Warming female tonic, enriches the blood, promotes blood circulation, regulates and normalizes menstruation and the menstrual cycle, mild laxative, diuretic, sedative, anti-inflammatory, analgesic, antibacterial, hypotensive, and antispasmodic.
- Dong quai, known for its therapeutic properties, offers a multifaceted approach to addressing a spectrum of gynecological concerns, from alleviating PMS symptoms to easing menopausal discomfort. Its effectiveness extends beyond the reproductive system, offering relief from ailments such as chronic pelvic infections and headaches attributed to blood deficiency.
- Also, its liver-supporting properties underscore a holistic approach to wellness, hinting at the intricate relationship between hormonal balance and hepatic function. Whether infused into a soothing tea or ingested in root form, the versatility of dong quai underscores its time-honored role in traditional herbal medicine.

ECHINACEA—Echinacea spp. in the Asteraceae or Aster family

Parts used: Root mostly, seeds, and flowers also
Taste/smell: The root is slightly sweet, pungent, aromatic, and tingles the tongue with most species.
Tendencies: Cooling, drying, stimulating

Uses:

- Antimicrobial, anti-inflammatory, antiviral, antibacterial, antifungal, slight stimulation of the adrenal cortex.
- Echinacea's dynamic role in immune support extends beyond its initial activation of white blood cells. Its efficacy lies not only in bolstering the body's natural defense mechanisms but also in its versatility as a remedy for various ailments. Whether applied topically to combat skin infections or internally to address digestive bacterial issues, echinacea's broad spectrum of applications underscores its significance as a potent herbal ally in maintaining overall health and well-being.

ELDERFLOWERS/BERRY—Sambucus spp. in the Caprifoliaceae or Honeysuckle family

Parts used: Flowers, berries
Taste/smell: Mucilaginous, slightly sweet
Tendencies: Cooling, drying

Uses:

- Expectorant, relaxing diaphoretic, diuretic, soothing nervine, mild laxative
- Elderflower/berry serves as a remedy for a range of conditions. In the early stages of coughs, colds, and flu, it has been historically employed, along with being effective against chronic sinusitis, spasmodic croup, night sweats, and skin eruptions due to metabolic disturbances. The juice extracted from its berries is particularly valued for its therapeutic properties, offering relief from

rheumatism, neuralgia, and common colds and flu. Elder flowers are considered suitable for children because they promote sweating and alleviate symptoms effectively.

ELECAMPANE—Inula helenium in the Asteraceae or Aster family

Parts used: Root
Taste/smell: Aromatic, pungent, sweet
Tendencies: Slightly warming, drying, stimulating

Uses:

- Antiseptic, expectorant, diaphoretic, bitter tonic, carminative, antiparasitic, anti-inflammatory, immunomodulating, diuretic, tonifying to the lungs and digestive system, strengthening, and cleansing to the respiratory tract mucous membranes.
- The elecampane herb has incredible healing potential for your lungs. Sometimes, it is recommended for lung rehabilitation. Most people use it when a cold is lasting too long, and they need to reach the deeper recesses of the bronchial tubes. It helps to remove phlegm from the respiratory tract and also works to heal the damaged lung tissue. Elecampane is strengthening and cleansing the respiratory tract mucous membranes. It is used for persistent bronchial catarrhs where there is an irritable cough, especially in chronic coughs of the elderly or invalid. It is specifically used for chronic bronchitis, sinusitis, tuberculosis, silicosis, moist asthma, and emphysema conditions. Elecampane assists with digestion and assimilation. It is used for gastroesophageal reflux and gastrointestinal ulcers.

ELEUTHERO/SIBERIAN GINSENG—Eleuthero coccus senticosus in the Araliaceae or Ginseng family

Part used: Root bark or cortex
Taste/smell: Bitter
Tendencies: Neutral to slightly warming

Uses:

- Adaptogen
- The Eleuthero root is also known as Siberian ginseng. It is distinct from Chinese ginseng and American ginseng. This root is considered neutral in terms of temperature, meaning it does not have the same heat-producing effects as the other types of ginsengs. Eleuthero is known for its stimulating properties and is more nourishing compared to other varieties of ginseng. It is commonly used to help balance immunity, mood, hormones, and stress levels. It has been used for centuries in traditional medicine for its adaptogenic properties, meaning it helps the body adapt to stress and supports overall resilience. Eleuthero root is prized for its ability to enhance the body's response to stress. It helps regulate the adrenal glands, which produce stress hormones like cortisol, and may improve the body's ability to cope with physical and mental stress. Eleuthero is often used to increase energy levels and stamina, making it popular among athletes and individuals seeking to enhance physical performance. It may also improve endurance and reduce fatigue.
- This herb is believed to strengthen the immune system, making it useful for preventing colds, flu, and other infections. It may help the body resist illness during times of increased stress or exposure to pathogens.
- Eleuthero root supports cognitive function, including memory, concentration, and mental clarity. It may help reduce mental fatigue and improve overall cognitive performance.

EYEBRIGHT—Euphrasia officinalis in the Scrophulariaceae or Figwort family

Parts used: Aerial parts
Taste/smell: Slightly bitter, slightly sweet
Tendencies: Drying

Uses:

- Astringent, expectorant, anti-inflammatory, antiseptic, decongestant
- Eyebright is good for eye conditions. It is believed to help reduce inflammation and soothe irritated mucous membranes. It's often used in herbal eye drops or washes to alleviate symptoms of conjunctivitis (both external and internal), as well as other eye irritations characterized by excessive tearing or discharge.
- In addition to its eye benefits, eyebright is also used for nasal congestion, sinusitis, and hay fever. Its astringent and anti-inflammatory properties make it useful for reducing nasal discharge and relieving sinus pressure.
- Eyebright can be prepared as an infusion for internal use or applied externally as compresses, eye drops, or nasal sprays. However, it's essential to consult with a healthcare professional before using eyebright or any herbal remedy, especially if you have underlying health conditions or are taking medication.

FENNEL—Foeniculum vulgare in the Apiaceae, previously Umbelliferae, or Parsley family

Parts used: Seed
Taste/smell: Aromatic, sweet, spicy
Tendencies: Warming

Uses:

- Mild expectorant
- Antispasmodic, thought to act on intestinal relaxation, uterus relaxation, bladder relaxation, anti-inflammatory, galactagogue, phytoestrogen, carminative, and flavoring

GARLIC (Allium sativum)

Parts used: Bulb
Taste/Smell: Pungent, spicy, sulfurous

Uses:

- Antimicrobial, immune support, cardiovascular health, reducing blood pressure, and cholesterol regulation.
- Garlic has been widely used in herbal medicine for its numerous health benefits. Rich in allicin, it is known for its antimicrobial, anti-inflammatory, and antioxidant properties. Garlic is commonly used to support cardiovascular health by lowering blood pressure and cholesterol levels. It is also believed to boost immunity, aid in digestion, and help combat infections like colds and flu. Additionally, garlic may have a role in managing blood sugar levels and promoting overall wellness.

GINGER (Zingiber officinale)

Parts used: Rhizome
Taste/Smell: Spicy, warm, aromatic

Uses:

- Anti-inflammatory, digestive aid, nausea relief, motion sickness, cold/flu remedy.
- Ginger is a popular herbal remedy valued for its anti-inflammatory, antioxidant, and digestive properties. It is commonly used to alleviate nausea, motion sickness, and indigestion. Ginger also helps reduce inflammation and pain, making it beneficial for conditions like arthritis. Its warming properties support circulation and immune health, and it may aid in managing colds, flu, and respiratory issues. Additionally, ginger has been studied for its potential to regulate blood sugar levels and support heart health.

GINGKO (Ginkgo biloba)

Parts used: Leaves, seeds
Taste/Smell: Mildly bitter (leaves), nutty (seeds)

Uses:

- Cognitive enhancement, memory support, circulation improvement, antioxidant properties.
- Ginkgo biloba is a widely used herbal remedy known for its potential to enhance brain function and improve memory. It is valued for its antioxidant and anti-inflammatory properties, which may support cognitive health and protect against age-related conditions like dementia. Ginkgo is also used to promote better blood circulation, particularly to the brain and extremities, and may help alleviate symptoms of conditions like tinnitus and vertigo. Additionally, it is believed to have benefits for managing anxiety and boosting overall mental clarity.

GOLDENSEAL (Hydrastis canadensis)

Parts used: Root, rhizome
Taste/Smell: Bitter, earthy

Uses:

- Antimicrobial, digestive aid, immune support, wound healing.
- Goldenseal is a versatile herbal remedy known for its antimicrobial and anti-inflammatory properties. Often used to support the immune system, it is commonly employed to address respiratory infections, digestive issues, and skin conditions. Goldenseal contains berberine, which may help combat bacteria, fungi, and viruses. It is also believed to soothe mucous membranes, making it beneficial for sore throats, sinusitis, and gastrointestinal discomfort. Additionally, goldenseal is used to promote liver health and overall detoxification.

GOOSEGRASS (Galium aparine)

Parts used: Whole plant
Taste/Smell: Mild, grassy

Uses:

- Detoxification, diuretic, lymphatic system support, skin conditions.
- Goosegrass, also known as cleavers or Galium aparine, is a traditional herbal remedy valued for its detoxifying and diuretic properties. It is commonly used to support lymphatic health, promoting the drainage of toxins and reducing swelling in conditions like lymphedema. Goosegrass is also believed to benefit the urinary system, helping to alleviate issues like urinary tract infections and kidney stones. Additionally, it has soothing properties that may aid in treating skin conditions such as eczema and psoriasis while supporting overall cleansing and wellness.

GOTU KOLA (Centella asiatica)

Parts used: Leaves, stems
Taste/Smell: Mild, earthy

Uses: Cognitive support, wound healing, skin health, stress reduction, and circulation improvement.

Gotu kola is a revered herb in traditional medicine, known for its ability to enhance brain function, promote wound healing, and improve circulation. It is often used to boost memory, focus, and mental clarity while reducing anxiety and stress. Gotu kola is also recognized for its skin-healing properties, aiding in the repair of wounds, burns, and scars. Additionally, it supports venous health, helping to alleviate varicose veins and improve blood flow. With its adaptogenic qualities, gotu kola is valued for promoting overall vitality and well-being.

GUARANA (Paulliniacupana)

Parts used: Seeds
Taste/Smell: Bitter, earthy

Uses: Stimulant, energy booster, mental focus, appetite suppressant.

Guarana (Paulliniacupana) is a popular herbal remedy known for its natural stimulant properties, primarily due to its high caffeine content. It is widely used to boost energy, enhance mental alertness, and combat fatigue. Guarana is also believed to support weight management by increasing metabolism and suppressing appetite. Additionally, it has antioxidant properties that may help reduce inflammation and protect against oxidative stress. Traditionally, guarana has been used to improve digestion, alleviate headaches, and promote cardiovascular health, making it a versatile natural tonic.

HIBISCUS (Hibiscus sabdariffa)

Parts Used: Flowers
Taste/Smell: Tart, floral, slightly sweet

Uses:

- Used in teas, jams, and beverages; supports heart health and the immune system; often used for its antioxidant properties.
- Hibiscus is a widely used herbal remedy known for its vibrant flowers and numerous health benefits. Rich in antioxidants, it helps combat oxidative stress and promotes heart health by lowering blood pressure and cholesterol levels. Hibiscus tea is commonly used to support digestion, aid in weight management, and regulate blood sugar levels. Its diuretic properties make it beneficial for reducing water retention and promoting kidney health. Additionally, hibiscus is celebrated for its immune-boosting and anti-inflammatory effects, making it a refreshing and healthful addition to a wellness routine.

HORSERADISH (Armoracia rusticana)

Parts Used: Root
Taste/Smell: Pungent, spicy, sharp

Uses:

- Used as a condiment, aids in digestion, promotes respiratory health, and has antibacterial properties.
- Horseradish is a potent herbal remedy valued for its antimicrobial and decongestant properties. It is commonly used to relieve sinus congestion, respiratory issues, and cold symptoms due to its natural ability to clear mucus and promote easier breathing. Rich in antioxidants, horseradish also supports immune health and helps combat infections. Its warming and stimulating properties may aid digestion, improve circulation, and provide relief from joint pain and inflammation. Additionally, horseradish has been traditionally used to support liver detoxification and overall vitality.

HOREHOUND (Marrubium vulgare)

Parts Used: Leaves, stems
Taste/Smell: Bitter, slightly minty

Uses:

- Used for coughs, colds, and respiratory issues; often found in cough syrups and lozenges.
- Horehound (Marrubium vulgare) is a traditional herbal remedy known for its effectiveness in treating respiratory and digestive ailments. It is commonly used as a natural expectorant to relieve coughs, soothe sore throats, and ease bronchial congestion. Horehound also supports digestion by stimulating bile production and alleviating symptoms like bloating and indigestion. Additionally, it has mild anti-inflammatory and antimicrobial properties, making it a valuable herb for addressing minor infections and promoting overall respiratory and gastrointestinal health.

HYSSOP (Hyssopus officinalis)

Parts Used: Leaves, flowers
Taste/Smell: Pungent, minty, slightly bitter

Uses:

- Used in digestive tonics, to treat respiratory issues, and as an antimicrobial; often used in aromatherapy.
- Hyssop (Hyssopus officinalis) is a versatile herb traditionally used for its respiratory and digestive benefits. Known for its expectorant properties, it helps relieve coughs, colds, and congestion by clearing mucus from the airways. Hyssop is also used to soothe sore throats and support overall respiratory health.
- In addition, it aids digestion by alleviating gas, bloating, and stomach discomfort. With mild antimicrobial and anti-inflammatory properties, hyssop can promote wound healing and support the immune system, making it a valuable addition to herbal remedies.

HOLY BASIL (*Ocimum sanctum* or *Ocimum tenuiflorum*)

Parts Used: Leaves, flowers
Taste/Smell: Spicy, clove-like, slightly sweet

Uses:

- Used in Ayurveda for stress relief, immune support, and anti-inflammatory purposes.
- Holy basil (Ocimum sanctum), also known as Tulsi, is a revered herb in traditional medicine, celebrated for its adaptogenic and therapeutic properties. It is commonly used to reduce stress, improve mental clarity, and promote emotional wellbeing. Holy basil is also known for its immune-boosting effects, helping to combat infections and support respiratory health. Its anti-inflammatory and antioxidant properties aid in reducing inflammation, protecting against oxidative stress, and supporting heart and metabolic health. Additionally, holy basil may help regulate blood sugar levels and promote overall vitality.

HELICHRYSUM (*Helichrysum italicum*)

Parts Used: Flowers
Taste/Smell: Sweet, slightly herbal, floral

Uses:

- Used in skincare for its anti-aging properties, reduces inflammation, and supports liver function.
- Helichrysum, often called "everlasting" or "immortelle," is a prized herb in traditional medicine, known for its powerful antiinflammatory, antioxidant, and skin-healing properties. It is commonly used to treat wounds, burns, and scars, promoting faster healing and tissue regeneration. Helichrysum is also valued for its ability to soothe respiratory conditions like coughs and congestion, as well as its potential to alleviate muscle and joint pain. Additionally, it supports overall skin health, helps reduce signs of aging, and is believed to aid in detoxification and emotional balance.

HOPS (*Humulus lupulus*)

Parts Used: Flowers (cones)
Taste/Smell: Bitter, floral, herbal

Uses:

- Commonly used in brewing beer; also used for relaxation, to reduce anxiety, and as a sleep aid.
- Hops (Humulus lupulus) are best known for their use in brewing beer, but they also have significant medicinal properties. Traditionally, hops are used as a natural sedative to promote relaxation, improve sleep quality, and reduce anxiety. Their bitter compounds support digestion by stimulating appetite and enhancing digestive enzyme production. Hops also have mild anti-inflammatory and antimicrobial properties, making them beneficial for soothing minor infections and discomfort. Additionally, they are believed to help balance hormones and alleviate symptoms of menopause, such ashot flashes and mood swings.

HEATHER (*Calluna vulgaris*)

Parts Used: Flowers, leaves
Taste/Smell: Mildly sweet, herbal, earthy

Uses:

- Used in teas and tinctures for urinary tract health, as an anti-inflammatory, and in skin care products.
- Heather (Calluna vulgaris) is a traditional herbal remedy known for its diuretic, anti-inflammatory, and soothing properties. It is commonly used to support urinary tract health, helping to alleviate conditions such as cystitis and kidney issues. Heather is also valued for its calming effects, making it useful in reducing stress and promoting relaxation. Additionally, its antiinflammatory properties can help soothe skin conditions like eczema and rashes. In traditional medicine, heather has been employed to support detoxification and overall wellness.

IRIS(Iris *germanica*)

Parts Used: Root
Taste/Smell: Earthy, sweet, floral

Uses:

- Used in traditional medicine for its diuretic and detoxifying properties, as well as in skincare for its soothing effects.
- Iris, particularly the root of the Orris variety (Iris germanica or Iris pallida), has been used in traditional herbal medicine for its aromatic and therapeutic properties. Orris root is known for its mild diuretic and expectorant effects, making it useful for
- supporting urinary health and relieving respiratory issues like coughs and congestion. It is also used in digestive remedies to alleviate bloating and promote better digestion. Additionally, iris is valued in skincare for its soothing and anti-inflammatory properties, often included in formulations to calm irritated or sensitive skin.

INDIAN GINSENG (*Withaniasomnifera*)

Parts Used: Root
Taste/Smell: Bitter, earthy

Uses:

- Known as Ashwagandha, it is used in Ayurvedic medicine for stress relief, energy boosting, and improving cognitive function.
- Indian ginseng, commonly known as Ashwagandha (Withaniasomnifera), is a powerful adaptogenic herb widely used in Ayurvedic medicine. It is renowned for its ability to reduce stress, improve energy levels, and enhance mental clarity. Ashwagandha supports the immune system, promotes restful sleep, and helps balance hormones, making it beneficial for overall vitality. It is also believed to improve strength and endurance, support cognitive function, and aid in managing conditions like anxiety, fatigue, and inflammation. Additionally, ashwagandha is often used to support reproductive health and promote a sense of well-being.

ICELAND MOSS (*Cetrariaislandica*)

Parts Used: Lichen
Taste/Smell: Slightly bitter, earthy

Uses:

- Used as a soothing agent for respiratory issues, coughs, and digestive complaints; also used in teas for its calming effects.
- Iceland moss (*Cetrariaislandica*) is a lichen traditionally used as a herbal remedy for its soothing and nourishing properties. Rich in mucilage, it is commonly used to relieve respiratory issues such as coughs, bronchitis, and throat irritation by coating and calming the mucous membranes. It also supports digestion by easing inflammation in the stomach and intestines, making it beneficial for conditions like gastritis and ulcers. Additionally, Iceland moss is valued for its mild antimicrobial and immune boosting properties, and it has historically been used as a nutrient-rich tonic during periods of recovery or malnutrition.

ITALIAN OREGANO (*Origanum vulgare hirtum*)

Parts Used: Leaves
Taste/Smell: Pungent, savory, slightly peppery

Uses:

- Used in cooking, particularly in Mediterranean dishes; known for its antimicrobial, antioxidant, and digestive properties.
- Italian oregano (*Origanum vulgare*), a staple in culinary and medicinal traditions, is valued for its potent antimicrobial, antioxidant, and anti-inflammatory properties. It is commonly used to support respiratory health, alleviating symptoms of colds, coughs, and sinus congestion. Oregano's strong antimicrobial compounds, such as carvacrol and thymol, make it effective in fighting bacterial, fungal, and viral infections. Additionally, it aids digestion by stimulating bile flow and reducing bloating. Italian oregano is also believed to

support immune health, promote overall detoxification, and protect against oxidative stress.

JAPANESE MINT (*Mentha canadensis*)

Parts Used: Leaves
Taste/Smell: Minty, cool, slightly sweet

Uses:

- Used in traditional medicine to relieve headaches, digestive issues, and muscle pain; also used in aromatherapy for relaxation.
- Japanese mint (*Mentha arvensis*), also known as cornmint, is a powerful herb widely used for its cooling and therapeutic properties. Rich in menthol, it is commonly employed to relieve respiratory conditions such as colds, congestion, and sinusitis by promoting clear airways. Japanese mint is also used to ease digestive issues like bloating, nausea, and indigestion. Its analgesic and anti-inflammatory properties make it effective for soothing headaches, muscle pain, and joint discomfort. Additionally, Japanese mint oil is often applied topically to invigorate and refresh the skin while promoting relaxation and mental clarity.

JASMINE (*Jasminum officinale*)

Parts Used: Flowers
Taste/Smell: Sweet, floral, fragrant

Uses:

- Used in aromatherapy for relaxation and stress relief; also used in teas for its soothing and mood-enhancing properties.
- Jasmine (*Jasminum spp.*) is a fragrant flowering plant valued in traditional medicine for its calming and uplifting properties. Known for its role in reducing stress, anxiety, and depression, jasmine is often used in aromatherapy to promote relaxation and emotional balance. Its antispasmodic properties make it helpful for easing

menstrual cramps and muscle tension. Jasmine is also believed to support digestive health and boost immunity with its mild antibacterial and anti-inflammatory effects. Additionally, jasmine tea is popular for its soothing qualities and potential to improve overall well-being.

JUNIPER (*Juniperus communis*)

Parts Used: Berries, needles
Taste/Smell: Piney, slightly sweet, aromatic

Uses:

- Used as a flavoring in cooking (especially in gin), for digestive health, and as a diuretic; also used in skin care for its cleansing properties.
- Juniper berries are aromatic seed cones used in culinary, medicinal, and spiritual practices. They add a piney, citrusy flavor to dishes, especially in European cuisine, and are essential in gin production. Traditionally, they aid digestion, support kidney health, and have antioxidant and anti-inflammatory properties. In aromatherapy and skincare, juniper berry oil is valued for its antibacterial and stress-relieving effects. Excessive consumption may be harmful, especially for pregnant women or those with kidney issues. Use in moderation.

KAVA (*Piper methysticum*)

Parts Used: Root
Taste/Smell: Earthy, bitter, slightly peppery

Uses:

- Used for its calming and sedative properties, helping with anxiety, stress, and insomnia. Often used in traditional Pacific Island ceremonies.
- Kava (*Piper methysticum*)is a traditional herb from the South Pacific known for its calming and relaxing effects. It is commonly used to reduce stress, anxiety, and tension while promoting a sense of

tranquility without impairing mental clarity. Kava is also valued for its ability to improve sleep quality, making it a popular natural remedy for insomnia. Additionally, it has mild analgesic and muscle-relaxant properties, which may help alleviate pain and muscle tension. Traditionally consumed as a drink, kava is celebrated for fostering social relaxation and emotional well-being.

KELP (*Ascophyllum nodosum* or *Laminaria spp.*)

Parts Used: Whole plant (often dried)
Taste/Smell: Salty, umami, oceanic

Uses:

- Used for its high iodine content, promoting thyroid health, as well as for its mineral and nutrient-rich properties, supporting detox and digestion.
- Kelp, a type of brown seaweed, is a nutrient-rich herbal remedy valued for its high content of iodine, vitamins, and minerals. It is commonly used to support thyroid health, as iodine is essential for proper thyroid hormone production. Kelp also promotes overall metabolic function, energy levels, and weight management. Rich in antioxidants, it helps combat oxidative stress and supports immune health. Additionally, kelp's fiber content aids digestion and may help regulate blood sugar levels. Its detoxifying properties are also believed to assist in removing heavy metals and toxins from the body.

KNOTWEED (*Polygonum multiflorum*)

Parts Used: Root
Taste/Smell: Earthy, bitter

Uses:

- Used in traditional Chinese medicine for anti-aging, supporting liver health, and boosting energy. Also known for its cardiovascular and antioxidant benefits.
- Knotweed, particularly Japanese knotweed (*Polygonum cuspidatum*), is a versatile herb known for its high concentration of resveratrol, a powerful antioxidant. It is commonly used to support cardiovascular health, promote circulation, and reduce inflammation. Knotweed is also valued for its ability to boost immune function and combat bacterial, viral, and fungal infections. In traditional medicine, it has been used to support joint health and alleviate conditions such as arthritis. Additionally, its antioxidant properties help protect against oxidative stress, making it a popular choice for promoting overall wellness and longevity.

KOREAN GINSENG (*Panax ginseng*)

Parts Used: Root
Taste/Smell: Bitter, earthy, slightly sweet

Uses:

- Known for its adaptogenic properties, helping to boost energy, improving cognitive function, and supporting the immune system.
- Korean ginseng (*Panax ginseng*), also known as red ginseng, is a powerful adaptogenic herb prized for its energy-boosting and stress-relieving properties. It is commonly used to enhance physical stamina, mental clarity, and overall vitality. Korean ginseng supports immune function, helps regulate blood sugar levels, and promotes cardiovascular health. It is also believed to improve cognitive function and memory, making it beneficial for brain health.

Additionally, it is used to enhance libido and reproductive health, as well as to support the body's natural resilience to stress and fatigue.

LAVENDER (Lavandula angustifolia)

Parts used: Flowers
Taste/Smell: Sweet, floral, slightly bitter

Uses:

- Calming, sleep aid, stress relief, skin healing, antimicrobial.
- Lavender (*Lavandula angustifolia*) is a widely cherished herb known for its calming and soothing properties. It is commonly used to reduce stress and anxiety, to promote restful sleep, often through aromatherapy or as an ingredient in herbal teas. Lavender also has anti-inflammatory and antimicrobial properties, making it effective for soothing skin irritations, minor burns, and insect bites. Additionally, it supports digestive health by alleviating bloating, indigestion, and nausea. With its gentle, versatile benefits, lavender is a favorite in natural remedies for relaxation, skincare, and overall well-being.

LEMON BALM (Melissa officinalis)

Parts used: Leaves
Taste/Smell: Citrusy, sweet

Uses:

- Anxiety relief, digestive aid, antiviral, improved focus, and sleep aid.
- Lemon balm (*Melissa officinalis*) is a fragrant herb known for its calming and uplifting effects. It is commonly used to reduce stress and anxiety and promote restful sleep. Lemon balm is also valued for its digestive benefits, helping to relieve indigestion, bloating, and nausea. With antiviral and antimicrobial properties, it supports immune health and has been traditionally used to alleviate cold sores and minor infections. Additionally, lemon balm is believed to

enhance focus and cognitive function, making it a versatile herb for promoting both relaxation and mental clarity.

LICORICE (Glycyrrhiza glabra)

Parts used: Root
Taste/Smell: Sweet, earthy

Uses:

- Respiratory health, soothing sore throat, digestive aid, anti-inflammatory.
- Licorice (Glycyrrhizaglabra) is a powerful herb used in traditional medicine for its soothing and healing properties. It is commonly used to alleviate respiratory issues like coughs, sore throats, and bronchitis due to its demulcent and anti-inflammatory effects. Licorice is also valued for supporting digestive health, helping to relieve symptoms of acid reflux, ulcers, and indigestion. Its adaptogenic properties aid in reducing stress and balancing cortisol levels. Additionally, licorice has antimicrobial and immune-boosting benefits, making it a versatile herb for promoting overall wellness.

LUNGWORT (Pulmonaria officinalis)

Parts used: Leaves
Taste/Smell: Mild, herbaceous

Uses:

- Respiratory support, cough relief, soothing irritated lungs.
- Lungwort (*Pulmonaria officinalis*) is a traditional herb known for its benefits in supporting respiratory health. It is commonly used to alleviate coughs, bronchitis, and other lung-related conditions due to its soothing and anti-inflammatory properties. Rich in mucilage, lungwort helps coat and protect the mucous membranes, easing irritation in the throat and airways. Additionally, it is believed to have mild antimicrobial effects, supporting the immune system in

fighting respiratory infections. Lungwort is also used to promote overall lung function and has been valued as a natural remedy for respiratory wellness.

LOVAGE (Levisticum officinale)

Parts used: Leaves, roots, seeds
Taste/Smell: Strong, celery-like

Uses:

- Digestive aid, diuretic, supports kidney health, flavoring agent.
- Lovage (*Levisticum officinale*) is a traditional herb valued for its diuretic, digestive, and anti-inflammatory properties. It is commonly used to support kidney and urinary tract health, helping to alleviate conditions like urinary tract infections and water retention. Lovage also aids digestion by reducing bloating, gas, and indigestion. Its expectorant properties make it beneficial for easing respiratory issues, such as coughs and congestion. Additionally, lovage has been used in traditional medicine to promote circulation, soothe joint discomfort, and support overall detoxification and wellness.

LADY'S MANTLE (Alchemilla vulgaris)

Parts used: Leaves, flowering tops
Taste/Smell: Astringent, slightly bitter

Uses:

- Menstrual support, wound healing, anti-inflammatory, digestive health.
- Lady's Mantle (*Alchemilla vulgaris*) is a traditional herb renowned for its benefits in women's health. It is commonly used to regulate menstrual cycles, ease menstrual cramps, and alleviate symptoms of menopause due to its astringent and hormone-balancing properties. Lady's Mantle also supports wound healing and helps soothe skin irritations, such as rashes and minor cuts. Its anti-inflammatory

and mild antibacterial effects make it useful for digestive health, helping to relieve diarrhea and gastrointestinal discomfort. This versatile herb is valued for its ability to promote overall wellness and hormonal balance.

LINDEN (Tilia spp.)

Parts used: Flowers, leaves
Taste/Smell: Sweet, floral

Uses:

- Relaxant, sleep aid, soothing colds and flu, mild diuretic.
- Linden (*Tilia spp.*), also known as lime flower, is a soothing herb widely used for its calming and therapeutic properties. It is commonly used to reduce stress and anxiety and promote restful sleep. Linden is also known for its ability to alleviate respiratory issues such as colds, coughs, and bronchitis, thanks to its soothing and expectorant effects. Additionally, linden supports heart health by promoting relaxation and improving circulation. Its mild diuretic and anti-inflammatory properties make it helpful for reducing fever, easing headaches, and soothing digestive discomfort, making it a versatile remedy in traditional herbal medicine.

LEMONGRASS (Cymbopogon citratus)

Parts used: Leaves, stalks
Taste/Smell: Citrusy, fresh

Uses:

- Digestive aid, stress relief, antimicrobial, flavoring in food and teas.
- Lemongrass (*Cymbopogon citratus*) is a fragrant herb widely used for its medicinal and culinary benefits. Known for its calming and digestive properties, it is commonly used to alleviate indigestion, bloating, and stomach cramps. Lemongrass is also valued for its antimicrobial and anti-inflammatory effects, making it useful in

supporting immune health and fighting infections. Additionally, it is believed to promote relaxation, reduce stress, and improve sleep. Lemongrass tea is a popular remedy for detoxification, while its essential oil is used in aromatherapy to uplift mood and invigorate the senses.

MARSHMALLOW (Althaea officinalis)

Parts used: Root, leaves, flowers
Taste/Smell: Mild, sweet, earthy

Uses:

- Soothing mucous membranes, cough relief, digestive health, skin irritation.
- Marshmallow (*Althaea officinalis*) is a soothing herb known for its high mucilage content, which provides protective and healing properties. It is commonly used to relieve irritation in the respiratory, digestive, and urinary systems. Marshmallow helps soothe sore throats, coughs, and bronchitis by coating mucous membranes. It is also effective in addressing digestive issues like acid reflux, ulcers, and gastritis. Additionally, marshmallow can ease urinary tract discomfort and support skin health by calming inflammation and promoting wound healing. This versatile herb is cherished for its gentle, soothing effects on the body.

MILK THISTLE (Silybum marianum)

Parts used: Seeds
Taste/Smell: Mild, slightly nutty

Uses:

- Liver support, detoxification, antioxidants, promotes lactation, supports digestive health.
- Milk thistle (*Silybum marianum*) is a renowned herb known for its liver-protective and detoxifying properties. The active compound, silymarin, is a powerful antioxidant that supports liver health by promoting regeneration of liver cells and protecting them from toxins and damage. Milk thistle is commonly used to treat liver conditions such as fatty liver disease, hepatitis, and cirrhosis. Additionally, it aids digestion, supports gallbladder health, and may help regulate blood sugar levels. It is also used by breastfeeding mothers to increase milk production. Its anti-inflammatory and antioxidant effects also make it beneficial for overall wellness and combating oxidative stress.

MEADOWSWEET (Filipendula ulmaria)

Parts used: Flowers, leaves
Taste/Smell: Sweet, slightly almond-like

Uses:

- Anti-inflammatory, digestive aid, supports joint health, fever relief.
- Meadowsweet (*Filipendula ulmaria*) is a traditional herb valued for its anti-inflammatory, pain-relieving, and digestive-supporting properties. It is commonly used to alleviate symptoms of acid reflux, indigestion, and stomach discomfort due to its gentle soothing effects on the digestive tract. Meadowsweet contains salicylates, making it effective for reducing fever, headaches, and joint pain associated with conditions like arthritis. Additionally, it has mild astringent and diuretic properties, which can support urinary health

and detoxification. This versatile herb is cherished for promoting comfort and overall well-being.

MINT (Mentha spp.)

Parts used: Leaves
Taste/Smell: Cool, refreshing, aromatic

Uses:

- Digestive aid, nausea relief, cooling, respiratory support.
- Mint (*Mentha spp.*) is a widely used herb known for its refreshing flavor and numerous health benefits. It is commonly used to support digestion, helping to relieve bloating, gas, and indigestion. Mint is also valued for its cooling and soothing properties, making it effective for easing headaches, nausea, and respiratory issues like congestion and coughs. Additionally, it has mild antimicrobial and anti-inflammatory effects, supporting oral health and soothing irritated skin. Mint's invigorating aroma is often used to reduce stress, boost focus, and promote a sense of well-being.

MORINGA (Moringa oleifera)

Parts used: Leaves, seeds, pods
Taste/Smell: Earthy, slightly bitter

Uses:

- Nutritional supplement, energy booster, immune support, anti-inflammatory.
- Moringa (*Moringa oleifera*), often called the "Drumstick tree" or
- "Miracle tree" is a nutrient-rich herb renowned for its wide-ranging health benefits. Packed with vitamins, minerals, antioxidants, and amino acids, it is commonly used to boost energy, enhance immunity, and support overall wellness. Moringa is known for its anti-inflammatory properties, making it beneficial for managing conditions like arthritis. It also supports heart health by helping to

regulate cholesterol and blood pressure levels and aids in blood sugar control. Additionally, moringa is used to promote healthy skin, improve digestion, and combat malnutrition, making it a versatile superfood in herbal medicine.

MOTHERWORT (Leonurus cardiaca)

Parts used: Aerial parts (leaves, flowers)
Taste/Smell: Bitter, earthy

Uses:

- Calming, supports heart health, stress relief, menstrual support.
- Motherwort (*Leonurus cardiaca*) is a traditional herb commonly used to support heart health and emotional well-being. Known for its calming properties, it is often used to reduce stress, anxiety, and symptoms of mild depression. Motherwort is also valued for its ability to regulate menstrual cycles, ease menstrual cramps, and alleviate symptoms of menopause. Its mild sedative and antispasmodic effects make it helpful for soothing nervous tension and promoting relaxation. Additionally, motherwort is believed to support cardiovascular health by helping to lower blood pressure and strengthen the heart, making it a popular choice in herbal medicine.

MULLEIN (Verbascum thapsus)

Parts used: Leaves, flowers
Taste/Smell: Mild, earthy

Uses:

- Respiratory support, soothing coughs, anti-inflammatory, supports ear health.
- Mullein (*Verbascum thapsus*) is a versatile herb known for its benefits in supporting respiratory health. It is commonly used to alleviate coughs, bronchitis, and asthma by soothing inflammation and

helping to clear mucus from the airways. Mullein's demulcent and expectorant properties make it effective for relieving sore throats and congestion. It is also valued for its mild antimicrobial and anti-inflammatory effects, supporting the immune system and overall lung health. Additionally, mullein can be used topically to soothe skin irritations and minor wounds, making it a staple in traditional herbal medicine.

MYRRH (Commiphora myrrha)

Parts used: Resin
Taste/Smell: Bitter, resinous, aromatic

Uses:

- Antimicrobial, wound healing, oral health, anti-inflammatory.
- Myrrh (*Commiphora myrrha*) is a resin widely valued in traditional medicine for its antimicrobial, anti-inflammatory, and healing properties. It is commonly used to support oral health, helping to alleviate gum infections, mouth ulcers, and sore throats. Myrrh is also known for its wound-healing abilities, making it effective for treating minor cuts, burns, and skin irritations. Additionally, it supports respiratory health by soothing coughs and congestion. Its antioxidant properties help combat oxidative stress, while its calming aroma is often used in aromatherapy to promote relaxation and spiritual grounding.

NETTLE (Urtica dioica)

Parts used: Leaves, roots, seeds
Taste/Smell: Earthy, slightly grassy

Uses:

- Nutrient-rich tonic, anti-inflammatory, supports allergies, kidney health, and hair growth.
- Nettle (*Urtica dioica*), also known as stinging nettle, is a nutrient-rich herb with a long history of use in traditional medicine. It is valued for its anti-inflammatory, diuretic, and antihistamine properties. Nettle is commonly used to support joint health, alleviate symptoms of arthritis, and reduce seasonal allergies like hay fever. Its diuretic effects make it beneficial for kidney and urinary health, helping to prevent and treat urinary tract infections. Rich in vitamins and minerals, nettle also supports energy levels, hair and skin health, and overall wellness. Additionally, it is used to promote detoxification and improve circulation.

NEEM (Azadirachta indica)

Parts used: Leaves, seeds, bark
Taste/Smell: Bitter, earthy

Uses:

- Antimicrobial, skin health, blood purification, immune support, insect repellent.
- Neem (*Azadirachta indica*) is a powerful herb widely used in traditional medicine for its antimicrobial, anti-inflammatory, and detoxifying properties. It is commonly employed to support skin health, treating conditions like acne, eczema, and psoriasis. Neem is also valued for its ability to boost immunity and combat bacterial, viral, and fungal infections. It is used to promote oral health, often in toothpaste or mouthwash, to reduce plaque and gum inflammation. Additionally, neem supports detoxification, liver health, and blood

sugar regulation, making it a versatile remedy for promoting overall well-being.

NIGHT-BLOOMING JASMINE (Cestrum nocturnum)

Parts used: Flowers, leaves
Taste/Smell: Sweet, aromatic

Uses:

- Soothing nerves, promoting sleep, and supporting respiratory health.
- Night-blooming jasmine (*Cestrum nocturnum*), also known as
- "Queen of the night" is a fragrant plant traditionally used in herbal medicine for its calming and medicinal properties. It is believed to support respiratory health, helping to alleviate coughs, asthma, and bronchitis due to its expectorant qualities. Additionally, night-blooming jasmine has been used to ease joint pain and inflammation in traditional remedies. Its calming scent is often utilized in aromatherapy to promote relaxation, reduce stress, and improve sleep. However, it should be used with caution, as parts of the plant can be toxic if ingested inlarge quantities.

NUTMEG (Myristica fragrans)

Parts used: Seed, mace (aril)
Taste/Smell: Warm, spicy, aromatic

Uses:

- Digestive aid, stress relief, supports sleep, anti-inflammatory.
- Nutmeg (*Myristica fragrans*) is a widely used spice with notable medicinal properties. It is valued for its digestive benefits, often used to relieve indigestion, bloating, and nausea. Nutmeg is also known for its calming effects, helping to reduce stress, promote relaxation, and improve sleep quality. Its anti-inflammatory and antioxidant properties support overall health and may help alleviate

joint pain. Additionally, nutmeg has been traditionally used to boost cognitive function and enhance focus. However, it should be consumed in moderation, as excessive intake can have toxic effects.

ONION (Allium cepa)

Parts used: Bulb, seeds
Taste/Smell: Pungent, sweet when cooked

Uses:

- Immune support, antimicrobial, cardiovascular health, digestive aid.
- Onion (*Allium cepa*) is a versatile vegetable with significant medicinal properties. Rich in antioxidants, particularly quercetin, it supports immune health and helps combat inflammation. Onions are commonly used to support cardiovascular health by improving blood circulation, reducing cholesterol levels, and lowering blood pressure. Their antimicrobial and expectorant properties make them effective in alleviating colds, coughs, and respiratory issues. Additionally, onions are believed to aid digestion, regulate blood sugar levels, and promote detoxification. They are a staple in both culinary and herbal traditions, valued for their health-boosting benefits.

OLIVE (Olea europaea)

Parts used: Leaves, fruit, oil
Taste/Smell: Bitter (leaves), rich and fruity (oil)

Uses:

- Antioxidant, cardiovascular support, immune booster, anti-inflammatory.
- Olive (*Olea europaea*), a staple of Mediterranean traditions, is renowned for its health-promoting properties. Olive leaves and oil are rich in antioxidants, particularly oleuropein, which support cardiovascular health by lowering blood pressure, improving

cholesterol levels, and protecting against oxidative stress. Olive oil is a cornerstone of a healthy diet, promoting brain health, reducing inflammation, andaidingin digestion. Olive leaf extracts are also valued for their antimicrobial and immuneboosting properties, helping to combat infections and support overall wellness. Additionally, olives are a good source of healthy fats, vitamins, and minerals that contribute to overall vitality.

ORRIS ROOT (Iris germanica)

Parts used: Root (rhizome)
Taste/Smell: Sweet, floral, violet-like aroma

Uses:

- Digestive support, respiratory health, used in perfumes and potpourri.
- Orrisroot, derived from the rhizomes of certain *Iris* species (such as *Iris germanica* or *Iris pallida*), is a fragrant herb traditionally used for its therapeutic and aromatic properties. It is often employed as a natural remedy to support digestive health, helping to alleviate bloating and indigestion. Orris root is also known for its mild diuretic effects, promoting kidney and urinary tract health. In addition, it has been used in oral care to freshen breath and maintain gum health. Its aromatic qualities make it a common ingredient in perfumes, powders, and potpourris.

OATSTRAW (Avena sativa)

Parts used: Aerial parts (stems, leaves), seeds
Taste/Smell: Mild, grassy

Uses:

- Nervous system support, calming, nourishing tonic, supports skin health.
- Oatstraw (*Avena sativa*) is a nourishing herb valued for its calming and restorative properties. Rich in vitamins, minerals, and antioxidants, it is commonly used to support nervous system health, reduce stress, and promote relaxation. Oatstraw is often employed to improve energy levels and combat fatigue without overstimulation. It also supports bone health due to its high calcium and silica content and aids in maintaining healthy skin and hair. Additionally, oatstraw is believed to have mild diuretic properties, promoting urinary health, and is cherished as a gentle, rejuvenating tonic for overall well-being.

PARSLEY (Petroselinum crispum)

Parts used: Leaves, stems, roots, seeds
Taste/Smell: Fresh, slightly peppery, earthy

Uses:

- Digestive aid, diuretic, detoxification, supports kidney and urinary health.
- Parsley (*Petroselinum crispum*) is a nutrient-rich herb widely used for its medicinal and culinary benefits. It is known for its diuretic properties, helping to support kidney and urinary health by reducing water retention and flushing out toxins. Rich in antioxidants like vitamin C and flavonoids, parsley supports immune health and helps combat inflammation. It is also a good source of vitamin K, which promotes bone health and proper blood clotting. Additionally, parsley aids digestion, freshens breath, and may help regulate blood sugar levels, making it a versatile and health-promoting herb.

PEPPERMINT (Mentha × piperita)

Parts used: Leaves
Taste/Smell: Cool, minty, aromatic

Uses:

- Digestive aid, nausea relief, respiratory support, headache relief.
- Peppermint (*Mentha × piperita*) is a versatile herb widely used for its soothing and refreshing properties. It is commonly employed to support digestive health, relieving symptoms of indigestion, bloating, and nausea. Peppermint's natural antispasmodic properties make it effective for easing muscle cramps and tension, including those associated with irritable bowel syndrome (IBS). Its cooling and decongestant effects are also beneficial for respiratory issues, such as colds, sinus congestion, and coughs. Additionally, peppermint is valued for its ability to improve focus, reduce stress, and alleviate headaches, making it a staple in both herbal medicine and aromatherapy.

PASSIONFLOWER (Passiflora incarnata)

Parts used: Leaves, flowers
Taste/Smell: Mild, grassy

Uses:

- Calming, sleep aid, stress relief, support nervous system health.
- Passionflower (*Passiflora incarnata*) is a calming herb known for its ability to reduce stress and anxiety and promote restful sleep. It is commonly used as a natural remedy for insomnia, helping to relax the mind and body without causing grogginess. Passionflower is also valued for its mild sedative and antispasmodic properties, making it effective for soothing nervous tension, muscle cramps, and digestive discomfort caused by stress. Additionally, it is believed to support heart health by lowering blood pressure and promoting relaxation, making it a popular choice for overall emotional and physical well-being.

PLANTAIN (Plantago major)

Parts used: Leaves, seeds
Taste/Smell: Mild, slightly earthy

Uses:

- Wound healing, soothing irritated skin, digestive aid, respiratory support.
- Plantain (*Plantago spp.*) is a versatile herb valued for its soothing and healing properties. It is commonly used to treat skin conditions such as wounds, insect bites, rashes, and burns due to its anti-inflammatory and antimicrobial effects. Rich in mucilage, plantain also soothes irritated mucous membranes, making it effective for alleviating coughs, sore throats, and digestive discomfort. Additionally, it is known for its ability to support urinary health and promote detoxification. Plantain is a popular choice in herbal medicine for its gentle yet powerful benefits in promoting healing and overall wellness.

PAPAYA (Carica papaya)

Parts used: Leaves, seeds, fruit
Taste/Smell: Sweet (fruit), slightly bitter (leaves)

Uses:

- Digestive aid, supports immune health, anti-inflammatory, wound healing.
- Papaya (*Carica papaya*) is a tropical fruit with significant medicinal properties. Rich in enzymes like papain and chymopapain, it is commonly used to aid digestion, relieve constipation, and reduce bloating. Papaya's anti-inflammatory properties make it beneficial for soothing conditions like arthritis and promoting
- wound healing. The fruit is packed with vitamins, antioxidants, and fiber, supporting immune health, skin regeneration, and heart health. Additionally, papaya seeds are known for their antimicrobial and detoxifying effects, often used to support liver health and

combat intestinal parasites, making the plant a versatile remedy for overall wellness.

PRICKLY ASH (Zanthoxylum spp.)

Parts used: Bark, berries
Taste/Smell: Spicy, pungent, numbing

Uses:

- Circulation improvement, digestive aid, supports nerve health, pain relief.
- Pricklyash (*Zanthoxylum spp.*), often called the "toothache tree," is a traditional herb known for its stimulating and warming properties. It is commonly used to support circulation, alleviate joint pain, and reduce numbness or tingling sensations. Prickly ash is also valued for its ability to relieve toothache and gum discomfort, thanks to its mild anesthetic effects. Additionally, it aids digestion by promoting the production of digestive enzymes and alleviating bloating or sluggish digestion. With its immune-boosting and detoxifying properties, prickly ash is a versatile herb in traditional herbal medicine.

PSYLLIUM (Plantago ovata)

Parts used: Seeds, husks
Taste/Smell: Mild, bland

Uses:

- Digestive health supports regular bowel movements and cholesterol regulation.
- Psyllium (*Plantago ovata*) is a highly effective herb known for its high fiber content and ability to support digestive health. Its seeds and husks act as a bulk-forming laxative, helping to relieve constipation and promote regular bowel movements by absorbing water and softening stool. Psyllium is also beneficial for managing diarrhea by

adding bulk to loose stools. Additionally, it supports heart health by lowering cholesterol levels and regulating blood sugar, making it useful for individuals with diabetes or metabolic concerns. Psyllium is a gentle, natural remedy widely used for maintaining digestive balance and overall wellness.

PINE (Pinus spp.)

Parts used: Needles, resin, bark
Taste/Smell: Resinous, piney

Uses:

- Respiratory support, antimicrobial, immune booster, supports circulation.
- Pine (*Pinus spp.*) is a versatile herb traditionally used for its respiratory, anti-inflammatory, and antimicrobial properties. The needles, bark, and resin are commonly employed to alleviate coughs, colds, bronchitis, and sinus congestion by clearing mucus and soothing the airways. Pine is also valued for its ability to relieve muscle pain and joint inflammation, often used in baths or as an essential oil in massage blends. Additionally, it has immune-boosting and antioxidant effects, supporting overall health. Pine preparations, such as teas or extracts, are cherished for their refreshing and revitalizing benefits.

QUASSIA (Quassia amara)

Parts used: Bark, wood
Taste/Smell: Extremely bitter, woody

Uses:

- Digestive aid, appetite stimulant, antiparasitic, antimicrobial.
- Quassia (*Quassia amara*or *Picrasma excelsa*) is a traditional herb valued for its bitter properties and various health benefits. It is commonly used to support digestion by stimulating appetite,

promoting the production of digestive enzymes, and alleviating indigestion or bloating. Quassia is also known for its antiparasitic properties, often used to treat intestinal worms and other parasitic infections. Additionally, it is believed to support liver health and help in detoxification. With antimicrobial and insecticidal properties, quassia is sometimes used in herbal formulations for skin conditions and as a natural pest repellent.

QUEEN ANNE'S LACE (Daucus carota)

Parts used: Seeds, roots
Taste/Smell: Earthy, slightly carrot-like

Uses:

- Diuretic, supports urinary health, menstrual regulation, digestive aid.
- Queen Anne's Lace (*Daucus carota*), also known as wild carrot, is a traditional herb valued for its diuretic and detoxifying properties. It is commonly used to support kidney and urinary tract health, helping to alleviate conditions such as water retention and bladder infections. The seeds of Queen Anne's Lace are also historically known for their use as a natural contraceptive in traditional medicine. Additionally, it supports digestive health and may help promote overall detoxification. However, caution is advised as it can be mistaken for toxic plants like poison hemlock. Proper identification is essential for safe use.

QUINCE (Cydonia oblonga)

Parts used: Fruit, seeds
Taste/Smell: Tart, fruity (fruit); bland, mucilaginous (seeds)

Uses:

- Digestive aid, soothing irritated mucous membranes, cough relief.
- Quince (*Cydonia oblonga*) is a fruit-bearing plant traditionally valued for its medicinal and nutritional benefits. Its fruit is rich in antioxidants, vitamins, and dietary fiber, supporting immune health, digestion, and overall wellness. Quince is commonly used to soothe digestive issues such as diarrhea and constipation due to its astringent and mucilage properties. Its anti-inflammatory effects make it helpful for relieving sore throats and soothing irritated skin when applied topically. Quince seeds are sometimes used in herbal remedies to create soothing gels for minor wounds and burns, making this plant a versatile addition to natural medicine.

ROSEMARY (Rosmarinus officinalis)

Parts used: Leaves, flowering tops
Taste/Smell: Piney, aromatic, slightly bitter

Uses:

- Cognitive support, digestive aid, circulatory stimulant, antioxidant.
- Rosemary (*Salvia rosmarinus*) is a fragrant herb renowned for its culinary and medicinal properties. It is commonly used to enhance memory, focus, and mental clarity, thanks to its circulation-boosting and antioxidant effects. Rosemary supports digestion by stimulating bile production and relieving indigestion or bloating. Its anti-inflammatory and antimicrobial properties make it effective for soothing sore muscles, improving scalp health, and promoting hair growth. Additionally, rosemary is believed to boost the immune system, improve circulation, and act as a natural mood enhancer, making it a versatile herb for both wellness and vitality.

RHUBARB (Rheum palmatum)

Parts used: Root (medicinal use), stalk (culinary use)
Taste/Smell: Bitter, astringent (root); tart (stalk)

Uses:

- Digestive health, laxative, liver support, anti-inflammatory.
- Rhubarb (*Rheum spp.*) is a versatile plant traditionally used for its digestive and medicinal benefits. The stalks are nutrient-rich and commonly consumed, while the roots are used in herbal medicine. Rhubarb root acts as a gentle laxative, helping to relieve constipation and support bowel regularity. It is also known for its astringent properties, which aid in managing diarrhea and promoting gastrointestinal health. Additionally, rhubarb contains antioxidants that support liver function and combat oxidative stress. However, caution is advised, as the leaves contain oxalic acid and are toxic if consumed.

RED CLOVER (Trifolium pratense)

Parts used: Flowers
Taste/Smell: Sweet, grassy

Uses:

- Hormonal balance, supports skin health, blood purification, and anti-inflammatory.
- Red clover (*Trifolium pratense*) is a nutrient-rich herb widely used for its medicinal properties, particularly in supporting women's health. It is rich in isoflavones, plant-based compounds that mimic estrogen, making it beneficial for alleviating symptoms of menopause, such as hot flashes and hormonal imbalances. Red clover is also valued for its detoxifying properties, supporting lymphatic health and promoting skin clarity. Additionally, it has anti-inflammatory and blood-thinning effects, which may support cardiovascular health. Traditionally, it is used to boost immune function and overall vitality, making it a versatile herb in natural medicine.

RUE (Ruta graveolens)

Parts used: Leaves, flowering tops
Taste/Smell: Bitter, strong, aromatic

Uses:

- Digestive aid, menstrual regulation, antimicrobial, insect repellent.
- Rue (*Ruta graveolens*) is a traditional herb valued for its antispasmodic, anti-inflammatory, and antimicrobial properties. It has been used to relieve menstrual cramps, promote regular menstruation, and support overall uterine health. Rue is also known for its ability to ease digestive discomfort, including bloating and gas, by stimulating bile production and aiding digestion. Additionally, it has been employed in folk medicine to alleviate joint pain, muscle spasms, and headaches. However, caution is necessary, as rue can be toxic in high doses and may cause skin irritation or adverse reactions if improperly used.

RASPBERRY (Rubus idaeus)

Parts used: Leaves, fruit
Taste/Smell: Mild, earthy (leaves); sweet and tart (fruit)

Uses:

- Menstrual and pregnancy support, digestive health, astringent, and antioxidant.
- Raspberry (Rubusidaeus), particularly its leaves, is a well-known herb in traditional medicine, valued for its astringent and nutritive properties. Raspberry leaf tea is commonly used to support women's reproductive health, helping to regulate menstrual cycles, ease menstrual cramps, and prepare the uterus for childbirth. It is also believed to promote smoother labor and recovery postpartum. Rich in vitamins and minerals, raspberry leaves support overall wellness, strengthen the immune system, and aid digestion. Additionally, its mild astringent effects make it useful for soothing diarrhea and inflammation in the digestive tract.

RHODIOLA (Rhodiola rosea)

Parts used: Root
Taste/Smell: Bitter, slightly floral

Uses:

- Adaptogen, stress relief, energy booster, cognitive support.
- Rhodiola (*Rhodiola rosea*), also known as Arctic root or golden root, is an adaptogenic herb prized for its ability to combat stress, fatigue, and mental exhaustion. It is commonly used to enhance energy levels, improve focus, and boost overall cognitive performance. Rhodiola is also believed to support physical endurance, making it popular among athletes and those with demanding lifestyles. Additionally, it has antioxidant properties that help protect against oxidative stress and support heart health. Rhodiola is a versatile herb that promotes resilience and balance, contributing to mental and physical well-being.

REISHI (Ganoderma lucidum)

Parts used: Fruiting body (mushroom)
Taste/Smell: Bitter, earthy

Uses:

- Immune support, stress reduction, sleep aid, anti-inflammatory.
- Reishi (*Ganoderma lucidum*), often called the "mushroom of immortality," is a revered medicinal fungus known for its immune-boosting, adaptogenic, and calming properties. It is commonly used to support overall immunity, helping the body combat infections and maintain balance. Reishi is also valued for its ability to reduce stress, improve sleep quality, and promote relaxation. With its anti-inflammatory and antioxidant effects, it supports heart health, liver function, and overall vitality. Additionally, reishi is believed to aid in managing fatigue, enhancing energy, and supporting longevity, making it a cornerstone in traditional and modern herbal medicine.

SAGE (Salvia officinalis)

Parts used: Leaves, flowering tops
Taste/Smell: Earthy, slightly bitter, aromatic

Uses:

- Digestive aid, cognitive support, antimicrobial, supports respiratory health.
- Sage (*Salvia officinalis*) is a highly regarded herb known for its medicinal and culinary uses. It is commonly used to support cognitive health and memory, often associated with its antioxidant and anti-inflammatory properties. Sage is also valued for its antimicrobial effects, making it effective for soothing sore throats, gum infections, and respiratory issues. It supports digestion by relieving bloating and indigestion and is believed to help regulate excessive sweating. Additionally, sage has been used to balance hormones, alleviate menopausal symptoms like hot flashes, and promote overall wellness, making it a versatile and beneficial herb.

ST. JOHN'S WORT (Hypericum perforatum)

Parts used: Leaves, flowering tops
Taste/Smell: Bitter, aromatic

Uses:

- Mood support, nerve health, wound healing, antiviral.
- St. John's Wort (*Hypericum perforatum) is a well-known herb primarily* used for its mood-enhancing properties. It is commonly employed to alleviate symptoms of mild to moderate depression, anxiety, and seasonal affective disorder (SAD) due to its active compounds, such as hypericin and hyperforin, which influence neurotransmitters in the brain. St. John's Wort also has anti-inflammatory, antimicrobial, and wound-healing properties, making it useful for treating minor cuts and burns. However, it can interact with medications, including antidepressants and birth control, so caution and medical advice are necessary before use.

SLIPPERY ELM (Ulmus rubra)

Parts used: Inner bark
Taste/Smell: Mild, slightly sweet, mucilaginous

Uses:

- Soothing mucous membranes, cough relief, digestive aid, and supporting irritated skin.
- Slippery elm (*Ulmus rubra*), derived from the inner bark of the tree, is a soothing herb valued for its high mucilage content. It is commonly used to alleviate irritation and inflammation in the digestive system, making it effective for conditions like acid reflux, gastritis, and irritable bowel syndrome (IBS). Slippery elm also soothes sore throats, coughs, and respiratory issues by coating mucous membranes. Additionally, it is used to promote healing in skin conditions such as wounds, burns, and eczema. Its gentle, demulcent properties make it a versatile remedy for both internal and external use.

SARSAPARILLA (Smilax spp.)

Parts used: Root
Taste/Smell: Earthy, slightly sweet

Uses:

- Blood purification, anti-inflammatory, supports skin health, detoxification.
- Sarsaparilla (*Smilax spp.*) is a traditional herb valued for its detoxifying, anti-inflammatory, and immune-boosting properties. It is commonly used to support skin health, helping to alleviate conditions like eczema, psoriasis, and acne. Sarsaparilla is also known for its blood-purifying effects, making it a popular choice in natural detoxification regimens. Additionally, it has been used to promote joint health, reduce inflammation, and improve symptoms of arthritis. Rich in plant compounds, such as saponins and

flavonoids, sarsaparilla supports liver and kidney health, enhances energy, and contributes to overall well-being.

SCHISANDRA (Schisandra chinensis)

Parts used: Berries
Taste/Smell: Sour, slightly sweet, bitter

Uses:

- Adaptogen, liver support, stress relief, enhances energy and endurance.
- Schisandra (*Schisandra chinensis*), often called the "five-flavor berry," is an adaptogenic herb prized for its ability to support overall health and resilience. It is commonly used to enhance energy, reduce stress, and improve mental clarity and focus. Schisandra is also known for its liver-protective properties, promoting detoxification and supporting healthy liver function. Additionally, it benefits respiratory health, boosts immunity, and provides antioxidant protection against oxidative stress. Schisandra is believed to promote hormonal balance, improve endurance, and contribute to longevity, making it a versatile herb in traditional and modern wellness practices.

STAR ANISE (Illicium verum)

Parts used: Fruit (seed pods)
Taste/Smell: Sweet, licorice-like, aromatic

Uses:

- Digestive aid, respiratory support, antimicrobial, flavoring agent.
- Star anise (*Illicium verum*) is a fragrant spice valued for its culinary and medicinal properties. Rich in shikimic acid, a compound used in antiviral medications, it is often employed to support immune health and combat respiratory infections like colds and flu. Star anise is also known for its carminative properties, helping to relieve

indigestion, bloating, and gas. Its antimicrobial and antifungal effects make it beneficial for overall health. Additionally, star anise is used to soothe coughs, promote relaxation, and enhance circulation, making it a versatile and warming remedy in traditional medicine.

SENNA (Senna alexandrina)

Parts used: Leaves, pods
Taste/Smell: Bitter, slightly grassy

Uses:

- Laxative, supports bowel health, detoxification.
- Senna (*Senna alexandrina*) is a well-known herbal remedy primarily used as a natural laxative. Its active compounds, called sennosides, stimulate the muscles of the colon, promoting bowel movements and relieving constipation. Senna is often used for short-term relief of occasional constipation or as part of bowel-cleansing regimens before medical procedures. It is also sometimes combined with other herbs to support overall digestive health. However, senna should be used with caution and not for extended periods, as overuse may lead to dependency or electrolyte imbalances. Proper dosage and medical guidance are recommended for safe use.

SPIRULINA (Arthrospira platensis)

Parts used: Whole algae
Taste/Smell: Earthy, sea-like

Uses:

- Nutritional supplement, energy booster, immune support, detoxification.
- Spirulina is a nutrient-dense blue-green algae renowned for its health benefits. Rich in protein, vitamins, minerals, and antioxidants, it is often used to boost energy, support the immune system, and

improve overall vitality. Spirulina is particularly valued for its anti-inflammatory properties, helping to combat oxidative stress and promote cardiovascular health. It also aids in detoxification, supporting liver function and helping to eliminate heavy metals from the body. Additionally, spirulina supports gut health, helps regulate blood sugar levels, and is a popular supplement for enhancing endurance and overall wellness.

SKULLCAP (Scutellarialateriflora)

Parts used: Leaves, flowering tops
Taste/Smell: Bitter, earthy

Uses:

- Calming, stress relief, nervous system support, sleep aid.
- Skullcap (Scutellaria spp.), particularly American skullcap (Scutellaria*lateriflora*), is a calming herb widely used to support the nervous system. It is commonly employed to reduce stress, anxiety, and nervous tension, promoting relaxation and emotional balance. Skullcap is also valued for its mild sedative properties, making it effective for improving sleep quality and alleviating insomnia. Additionally, it has anti-inflammatory and antioxidant effects, which may help support brain health and protect against oxidative stress. Skullcap is a gentle yet powerful remedy for promoting mental clarity, calmness, and overall well-being.

SHEPHERD'S PURSE (Capsella bursa-pastoris)

Parts used: Aerial parts
Taste/Smell: Mild, slightly peppery

Uses:

- Stops bleeding, menstrual support, supports urinary health, wound healing.
- Shepherd's purse (*Capsella bursa-pastoris*) is a traditional herb known for its astringent and styptic properties, making it effective in reducing bleeding. It is commonly used to address heavy menstrual bleeding, postpartum hemorrhage, and other bleeding conditions. Shepherd's purse is also valued for its ability to support wound healing and alleviate inflammation. Additionally, it has diuretic properties, which may aid in treating urinary tract issues and reducing water retention. This versatile herb is often used to promote overall circulatory and reproductive health, particularly in managing bleeding-related concerns.

THYME (Thymus vulgaris)

Parts used: Leaves, flowering tops
Taste/Smell: Earthy, aromatic, slightly peppery

Uses:

- Antimicrobial, respiratory support, digestive aid, antioxidant.
- Thyme (*Thymus vulgaris*) is a versatile herb known for its antimicrobial, antioxidant, and anti-inflammatory properties. It is commonly used to support respiratory health, helping to alleviate coughs, bronchitis, and congestion by loosening mucus and soothing the airways. Thyme also aids digestion by reducing bloating and promoting the breakdown of fats. Its antiseptic qualities make it useful for treating minor wounds and supporting oral health, such as combating gum infections and bad breath. Additionally, thyme boosts the immune system, fights infections, and promotes

overall wellness, making it a staple in both culinary and medicinal traditions.

TURMERIC (Curcuma longa)

Parts used: Rhizome
Taste/Smell: Earthy, slightly bitter, warm

Uses:

- Anti-inflammatory, antioxidant, supports joint health, liver support, immune booster.
- Turmeric (*Curcuma longa*) is a powerful herb widely valued for its anti-inflammatory, antioxidant, and healing properties. Its active compound, curcumin, is known for supporting joint health, alleviating arthritis symptoms, and reducing inflammation throughout the body. Turmeric is also used to enhance digestion, support liver detoxification, and promote heart health by improving cholesterol levels and circulation. Additionally, it boosts the immune system and may help combat oxidative stress, potentially reducing the risk of chronic diseases. Turmeric is a versatile herb used in traditional and modern medicine to promote overall wellness and vitality.

TULSI (Ocimum sanctum)

Parts used: Leaves, flowering tops
Taste/Smell: Sweet, spicy, aromatic

Uses:

- Adaptogen, stress relief, immune support, respiratory health, digestive aid.
- Tulsi (*Ocimum sanctum* or *Ocimum tenuiflorum*), also known as Holy Basil, is a revered herb in Ayurvedic medicine, celebrated for its adaptogenic and healing properties. It is commonly used to reduce stress, enhance mental clarity, and promote emotional balance.

Tulsi supports respiratory health, helping to alleviate colds, coughs, and asthma, while also boosting the immune system. Its anti-inflammatory and antioxidant properties protect against oxidative stress and support heart health. Additionally, Tulsi aids digestion, regulates blood sugar levels, and promotes overall detoxification, making it a cornerstone in natural wellness practices.

TEA TREE

Parts used: Leaves, stems
Taste/Smell: Sweet, anise-like, slightly peppery

Uses:

- treat acne, athlete's foot, lice, fungus, and insect bites.
- Tea tree (*Melaleuca alternifolia*) is a highly valued medicinal plant known for its potent antimicrobial, antifungal, and anti-inflammatory properties. Its essential oil is widely used to treat skin conditions such as acne, eczema, and fungal infections like athlete's foot. Tea tree oil is also effective for soothing minor cuts, insect bites, and burns due to its antiseptic qualities. Additionally, it is used in oral care products to combat bad breath and gum infections and in hair care to address dandruff and scalp irritation. Highly versatile, tea tree is a staple in natural remedies and skincare.

TARRAGON (Artemisia dracunculus)

Parts used: Leaves, stems
Taste/Smell: Sweet, anise-like, slightly peppery

Uses:

- Digestive aid, appetite stimulant, supports cardiovascular health, antioxidant.
- Tarragon (*Artemisia dracunculus*), a fragrant herb commonly used in culinary traditions, also holds medicinal value. It is known for its ability to support digestive health, helping to stimulate appetite and

alleviate indigestion, bloating, and stomach discomfort. Tarragon contains compounds with mild sedative properties, making it useful for promoting relaxation and improving sleep. It is also believed to support cardiovascular health and regulate blood sugar levels. Rich in antioxidants, tarragon helps combat oxidative stress, contributing to overall wellness. Its blend of flavor and health benefits makes it a valuable herb in both food and traditional remedies.

TIGER NUT (Cyperus esculentus)

Parts used: Tubers
Taste/Smell: Sweet, nutty

Uses:

- Digestive health, energy booster, supports blood sugar regulation, nutrient-rich tonic.
- Tiger nut (*Cyperus esculentus*), a nutrient-rich tuber, is known for its health benefits and versatility. High in dietary fiber, it supports digestive health by promoting regular bowel movements and improving gut microbiota. Tiger nuts are also a natural source of resistant starch, which aids in blood sugar regulation and provides sustained energy. Rich in healthy fats, vitamins, and minerals like magnesium and potassium, they contribute to heart health and overall vitality. Additionally, tiger nuts are gluten-free and lactose-free, making them a popular choice for those with dietary restrictions. Their sweet, nutty flavor and nutritional value make them a valuable addition to both traditional and modern diets.

TRIBULUS (Tribulus terrestris)

Parts used: Fruits, roots
Taste/Smell: Bitter, earthy

Uses:

- Hormonal balance, energy booster, supports reproductive health, anti-inflammatory.
- Tribulus (*Tribulus terrestris*), commonly known as puncture vine, is a herb widely used in traditional medicine for its potential to enhance vitality and overall wellness. It is commonly employed to support reproductive health, often associated with boosting libido, improving fertility, and balancing hormones in both men and women. Tribulus is also believed to promote muscle strength and endurance, making it popular among athletes and fitness enthusiasts. Additionally, it has diuretic properties that may support urinary health and aid in detoxification. Rich in antioxidants, Tribulus also helps combat oxidative stress and supports cardiovascular health.

ULMUS (Ulmus rubra)

Parts used: Inner bark
Taste/Smell: Mild, slightly sweet, mucilaginous

Uses:

- Soothing mucous membranes, digestive health, cough relief, skin support.
- *Ulmus*, commonly known as slippery elm (*Ulmus rubra*), is a tree valued for its medicinal inner bark, which has soothing and healing properties. Rich in mucilage, slippery elm is used to coat and protect irritated mucous membranes, making it effective for relieving sore throats, coughs, and respiratory discomfort. It is also a popular remedy for digestive issues such as acid reflux, gastritis, and irritable bowel syndrome (IBS). Additionally, slippery elm aids in soothing urinary tract irritation and promoting wound healing when

applied topically. Its gentle, demulcent effects make it a staple in traditional herbal medicine.

UVA URSI (Arctostaphylos uva-ursi)

Parts used: Leaves
Taste/Smell: Bitter, astringent

Uses:

- Traditionally used to support urinary tract health, as a diuretic, and to help manage bladder infections. It has antimicrobial properties and is often used for conditions like cystitis and urethritis.
- Uva ursi (*Arctostaphylos uva-ursi*), also known as bearberry, is a traditional herb valued for its ability to support urinary tract health. It is commonly used to alleviate urinary tract infections (UTIs) and bladder inflammation due to its antimicrobial and astringent properties. The active compound, arbutin, converts to hydroquinone in the body, providing antibacterial effects within the urinary tract. Uva ursi is also a natural diuretic, helping to flush out bacteria and toxins. However, it is recommended for short-term use and should be used with caution under professional guidance, as prolonged or excessive use may have adverse effects.

VALERIAN (Valeriana officinalis)

Parts used: Root, rhizome
Taste/Smell: Earthy, musky, slightly bitter

Uses:

- Calming, sleep aid, stress relief, supports nervous system health.
- Valerian (*Valeriana officinalis*) is a well-known herb traditionally used for its calming and sedative properties. It is commonly employed to promote restful sleep, alleviate insomnia, and reduce anxiety and stress. Valerian works by influencing the nervous system, helping to relax the mind and body without causing grogginess. Additionally, it

is used to relieve muscle tension, menstrual cramps, and headaches due to its antispasmodic effects. Valerian is a popular natural remedy for improving emotional balance, soothing nervous tension, and supporting overall relaxation and well-being.

VERVAIN (Verbena officinalis)

Parts used: Leaves, flowering tops
Taste/Smell: Bitter, slightly astringent

Uses:

- Nervous system support, digestive aid, supports mood balance, promotes relaxation.
- Vervain (*Verbena officinalis*), also known as common vervain, is a traditional herb prized for its calming and restorative properties. It is commonly used to reduce stress, anxiety, and mild depression, promoting emotional balance and relaxation.
- Vervain is also valued for its ability to support digestion, relieve bloating, and stimulate appetite. Known for its anti-inflammatory and mild analgesic effects, it has been used to ease headaches, menstrual discomfort, and muscle tension. Additionally, vervain is believed to support liver health and detoxification, making it a versatile herb in traditional herbal medicine.

VIOLET (Viola odorata)

Parts used: Leaves, flowers
Taste/Smell: Sweet, mild, slightly grassy

Uses:

- Respiratory support, soothing mucous membranes, skin health, mild laxative.
- Violet (*Viola odorata*), also known as sweet violet, is a delicate herb with soothing and medicinal properties. It is commonly used to support respiratory health, helping to relieve coughs, colds, and

bronchitis by soothing irritation and promoting mucus clearance. Violet is also valued for its anti-inflammatory and antioxidant effects, making it beneficial for skin conditions like eczema, acne, and minor wounds. Additionally, it is believed to aid in detoxification, support lymphatic health, and promote relaxation. Violet leaves and flowers are gentle yet effective, making them a cherished remedy in traditional herbal practices.

VANILLA (Vanilla planifolia)

Parts used: Pods (beans)
Taste/Smell: Sweet, warm, aromatic

Uses:

- Flavoring agent, supports mood, antioxidant, mild aphrodisiac.
- Vanilla (*Vanilla planifolia*) is a fragrant and flavorful herb widely appreciated for its culinary and medicinal properties. Its primary active compound, vanillin, is known for its antioxidant and anti-inflammatory effects, which help combat oxidative stress and support overall wellness. Vanilla is often used in aromatherapy to promote relaxation, reduce stress, and enhance mood. It may also aid digestion and soothe an upset stomach. Additionally, vanilla has mild antimicrobial properties and is sometimes used in natural skincare to nourish and protect the skin. Its comforting aroma and versatile benefits make it a popular choice in traditional and modern remedies.

VIBURNUM (Viburnum opulus)

Parts used: Bark, berries
Taste/Smell: Bitter, slightly astringent

Uses:

- Muscle relaxant, menstrual support, supports uterine health, anti-inflammatory.
- Viburnum, particularly species like *Viburnum opulus*(cramp bark) and *Viburnum prunifolium*(black haw), is a traditional herb known for its antispasmodic and calming properties. It is commonly used to relieve menstrual cramps, uterine spasms, and discomfort associated with PMS. Viburnum is also valued for its ability to ease muscle tension and support relaxation. In traditional medicine, it is used to support reproductive health, particularly for reducing the risk of miscarriage and promoting smooth labor. Additionally, its anti-inflammatory and astringent properties make it beneficial for addressing joint pain and digestive discomfort.

WORMWOOD (Artemisia absinthium)

Parts used: Leaves, flowering tops
Taste/Smell: Bitter, aromatic

Uses:

- Digestive aid, antiparasitic, supports liver health, appetite stimulant.
- Wormwood (*Artemisia absinthium*) is a potent herb traditionally used for its antiparasitic, antimicrobial, and digestive properties. It is commonly employed to treat intestinal worms and other parasitic infections. Wormwood also supports digestion by stimulating bile production, relieving bloating, and enhancing appetite. Its anti-inflammatory and antioxidant properties make it useful for addressing joint pain and inflammation. Additionally, wormwood is a key ingredient in absinthe and herbal bitters, valued for promoting gastrointestinal health. However, caution is necessary as excessive

use can be toxic due to its thujone content, so it should be used under professional guidance.

WHITE WILLOW (Salix alba)

Parts used: Bark
Taste/Smell: Bitter, earthy

Uses:

- Pain relief, anti-inflammatory, supports joint health, fever reduction.
- White willow (*Salix alba*) is a traditional herb renowned for its natural pain-relieving and anti-inflammatory properties. Its bark contains salicin, a compound that the body converts to salicylic acid, making it a natural precursor to aspirin. White willow is commonly used to alleviate headaches, muscle pain, arthritis, and menstrual cramps. Additionally, it is valued for its ability to reduce fever and soothe inflammation. With antioxidant properties, white willow supports overall wellness. It is a gentle yet effective remedy, often preferred as a natural alternative to synthetic pain relievers, though it should be used with caution in individuals sensitive to salicylates.

WATERCRESS (Nasturtium officinale)

Parts used: Leaves, stems
Taste/Smell: Peppery, slightly tangy

Uses:

- Digestive health, nutrient-rich tonic, supports respiratory health, detoxification.
- Watercress (*Nasturtium officinale*) is a nutrient-dense herb known for its detoxifying and health-promoting properties. Rich in vitamins A, C, and K, as well as minerals like calcium and iron, it supports bone health, boosts immunity, and promotes overall vitality. Watercress is also valued for its antioxidant properties, helping to combat oxidative stress and reduce inflammation. Traditionally, it

has been used to support respiratory health, digestion, and liver detoxification. Its diuretic effects aid in flushing out toxins, while its slightly peppery flavor makes it a popular addition to both culinary and herbal practices.

WINTERGREEN (Gaultheria procumbens)

Parts used: Leaves
Taste/Smell: Minty, aromatic

Uses:

- Pain relief, anti-inflammatory, supports joint health, flavoring agent.
- Wintergreen (*Gaultheria procumbens*) is a fragrant herb known for its natural pain-relieving and anti-inflammatory properties. Its leaves contain methyl salicylate, a compound similar to aspirin, making it effective for soothing muscle aches, joint pain, and arthritis. Wintergreen is often used in topical applications, such as oils, balms, and liniments, to provide relief from pain and stiffness. Additionally, it has mild antimicrobial and astringent properties, supporting oral health and helping to alleviate sore throats. While highly beneficial externally, internal use of wintergreen requires caution due to its potent nature.

WITCH HAZEL (Hamamelis virginiana)

Parts used: Bark, leaves
Taste/Smell: Astringent, slightly woody

Uses:

- Skin health, wound healing, anti-inflammatory, soothes irritation.
- Witch hazel (*Hamamelis virginiana*) is a widely used herb known for its astringent and anti-inflammatory properties. Extracts from its bark and leaves are commonly applied topically to soothe skin irritations, reduce swelling, and promote healing of conditions such as acne, eczema, and minor cuts or burns. Witch hazel is

also effective in relieving hemorrhoids and varicose veins by reducing inflammation and improving circulation. Additionally, its antimicrobial properties make it useful for cleansing wounds and preventing infection. Gentle yet effective, witch hazel is a staple in natural skincare and first-aid remedies.

WILD YAM (Dioscorea villosa)

Parts used: Root, rhizome
Taste/Smell: Earthy, slightly bitter

Uses:

- Hormonal balance, menstrual support, anti-inflammatory, supports joint health.
- Wild yam (*Dioscorea villosa*) is a traditional herb valued for its potential to support hormonal and reproductive health. It is commonly used to alleviate menstrual cramps, premenstrual syndrome (PMS), and menopausal symptoms, such as hot flashes and mood swings. Wild yam is also believed to have antispasmodic properties, making it effective for soothing muscle spasms and digestive discomfort. Additionally, it has been used in herbal medicine to support joint health and reduce inflammation. While sometimes associated with natural hormone replacement therapy, further research is needed to fully understand its hormonal effects.

WOOD BETONY (Stachys officinalis)

Parts used: Leaves, flowering tops
Taste/Smell: Mild, slightly bitter, earthy

Uses:

- Nervous system support, digestive aid, headache relief, and promotes relaxation.
- Wood betony (*Stachys officinalis*), also known as betony, is a traditional herb valued for its calming and restorative properties. It is commonly used to support nervous system health, helping to relieve stress, anxiety, and headaches. Wood betony is also known for its ability to ease digestive discomfort, including bloating and indigestion, and to support liver function. Additionally, it has mild anti-inflammatory and astringent properties, making it helpful for soothing sore throats and minor wounds. With a long history in herbal medicine, wood betony is cherished for promoting relaxation and overall well-being.

YARROW (Achillea millefolium)

Parts used: Leaves, flowers
Taste/Smell: Bitter, astringent, slightly aromatic

Uses:

- Wound healing, fever reduction, digestive aid, menstrual support, anti-inflammatory.
- Yarrow (*Achillea millefolium*) is a versatile herb known for its astringent, anti-inflammatory, and healing properties. It is commonly used to stop bleeding, both internally and externally, and to promote wound healing. Yarrow supports digestive health by alleviating bloating, indigestion, and cramps, while its antispasmodic properties make it effective for menstrual discomfort. It is also valued for its ability to reduce fever and support respiratory health by easing congestion and soothing colds. Additionally, yarrow has

mild antimicrobial properties and is often used to support the immune system and overall wellness.

YOHIMBE (Pausinystaliajohimbe)

Parts used: Bark
Taste/Smell: Bitter, earthy

Uses:

- Supports circulation, aphrodisiac, energy booster, used for erectile dysfunction.
- Yohimbe (*Pausinystaliajohimbe*) is a traditional herb derived from the bark of an African tree, known for its stimulant and aphrodisiac properties. It is commonly used to support sexual health, particularly to improve erectile function and enhance libido in men and women. Yohimbe is also believed to promote energy, improve athletic performance, and support weight loss by increasing metabolism and blood flow. However, caution is necessary, as yohimbe can cause side effects such as increased heart rate, anxiety, and high blood pressure if taken in excess. Its use should be guided by a healthcare professional.

YELLOW DOCK (Rumex crispus)

Parts used: Root
Taste/Smell: Bitter, earthy

Uses:

- Detoxification, supports liver health, digestive aid, mild laxative, promotes skin health.
- Yellow dock (*Rumex crispus*) is a traditional herb valued for its detoxifying and nourishing properties. It is commonly used to support liver and kidney health, aiding in the removal of toxins and promoting overall detoxification. Yellow dock is also known for its mild laxative effects, making it helpful for relieving constipation

and supporting digestive health. Rich in iron and minerals, it is often used to address anemia and improve skin conditions such as eczema, psoriasis, and acne. Additionally, its anti-inflammatory and antimicrobial properties make it a versatile remedy for promoting overall wellness.

YERBA MATE (Ilex paraguariensis)

Parts used: Leaves, stems
Taste/Smell: Earthy, slightly bitter, smoky

Uses:

- Energy booster, antioxidant, supports focus and mental clarity, mild diuretic.
- Yerba mate (*Ilex paraguariensis*) is a stimulating herb traditionally consumed as a tea in South America, renowned for its energizing and health-boosting properties. It is rich in antioxidants, vitamins, and minerals, making it a powerful supporter of overall wellness. Yerba mate is commonly used to enhance mental focus, boost energy levels, and improve physical performance. It also aids digestion, supports weight management by promoting fat oxidation and reducing appetite, and helps regulate blood sugar levels. Additionally, its anti-inflammatory and immune-enhancing properties make it a popular choice for promoting vitality and well-being.

YUCCA (Yucca schidigera)

Parts used: Root, stem
Taste/Smell: Mild, slightly earthy

Uses:

- Anti-inflammatory, supports joint health, digestive aid, used in skin and hair products.
- Yucca (*Yucca spp.*) is a desert plant traditionally used for its anti-inflammatory and antioxidant properties. It is commonly employed to support joint health and alleviate symptoms of arthritis and other inflammatory conditions. Yucca contains saponins, which may aid in reducing swelling and promoting overall comfort. Additionally, it supports digestive health by improving nutrient absorption and aiding in detoxification. Yucca is also valued for its potential to boost skin health, help with hair growth, and promote overall vitality. Its versatile benefits make it a staple in traditional medicine for promoting wellness and managing inflammation.

ZIZIPHUS (Ziziphus jujuba)

Parts used: Fruits, seeds
Taste/Smell: Sweet (fruit), mild and nutty (seeds)

Uses:

- Supports sleep, stress relief, digestive aid, and promotes skin health.
- Ziziphus (*Ziziphus jujuba*), commonly known as jujube or Chinese date, is a traditional herb widely valued for its calming and restorative properties. It is often used to alleviate stress, promote relaxation, and improve sleep quality. Rich in antioxidants, vitamins, and minerals, Ziziphus supports immune health, protects against oxidative stress, and promotes overall vitality. It is also believed to aid digestion, improve circulation, and support heart health. In traditional medicine, Ziziphus is cherished for its ability to nourish the body and mind, making it a versatile remedy for enhancing overall well-being.

ZINCWORT (Gypsophila spp.)

Parts used: Root
Taste/Smell: Bitter, slightly soapy

Uses:

- Supports respiratory health, used as a natural soap (saponins), aids in detoxification.
- Zincwort is a less commonly known herb, but it often refers to plants like *Spergularia rubra*, traditionally used for their medicinal properties. It is valued for its diuretic and detoxifying effects, making it useful for supporting kidney and urinary tract health. Zincwort has been used in traditional remedies to help alleviate water retention, cleanse the body of toxins, and support skin health. Its gentle action makes it a candidate for herbal preparations aimed at overall detoxification and wellness. However, specific details about its active compounds and modern applications may vary, so professional guidance is recommended for its use.

2

Types of preparations and uses

Capsules

Most people find capsules to be convenient, easy, and better for traveling. When you take the capsules, you have no taste, and that seems to be a big plus for a lot of people. Also, since the supplement market is now so huge, taking capsules and tablets is now seen as normal and widely accepted. They are easier for people to keep around than herbal tinctures and salves.

Even though capsules and tablets are easy to transport, and they are very accessible, they are not always the best option for you. A person who has a digestive imbalance, for example, may not be able to reap the full benefits if they already have the inability to break food down properly. For these people, I would encourage you to consider other modes of medicine transmission when the digestive system has been challenged.

One thing is certain, though: herbal capsules are very easy to make. Using herbal powder makes the whole process much easier and quicker. You can grind the dried-up herbs with an herb grinder, or you can purchase the herb powder already prepared. There are two capsule materials to choose from: gelatin and vegetable glycerin. Gelatin may be cheaper, but most people prefer the natural vegetable glycerin capsules. The empty capsules come in different sizes starting from 0 (the smallest), 00, and 000 (the largest).

Essential Oil Blends

Essential oils can be blended together, added to another herbal formula, or used in another way that plants can provide healing for you. Essential oils are derived through extraction by using one of the following methods: water distillation, solvent extraction, cold press extraction, steam distillation, or CO_2 extraction. The methods listed pull out the oils from the plant, and most of them will yield both essential oil and water. The essential oil will sit on top of the water. After processing, this is called a hydrosol. This rich oil contains specific medicinal constituents, and the hydrosol has medicinal properties as well, but these are typically limited to the water-soluble aspects of the plant.

You will find that some of the recipes in this book will direct you to add some essential oils to other ingredients to make salves or herbal oils, and other recipes will tell you how to create essential oil blends that target specific health conditions. For the blends that consist of only essential oils, the essential oil quantity is indicated in milliliters, since the typical essential oil bottle is 5 or 10 milliliters. If the essential oil recipe asks for you to use a carrier oil, the measurements are in drops of essential oil and in ounces of the carrier oil.

It is recommended to always use pure therapeutic essential oils with your healing recipes. Be sure to keep the caps on the bottles tightly. A pure essential oil is capable of evaporating if the cap is left off. Essential oils can be used in many ways, but I do not recommend applying them directly to your skin because it can be quite caustic, or in other words, it could burn your skin.

If you wish to use an essential oil topically on your skin, you should first dilute it with apricot, olive, or coconut oil. Some essential oils, especially oregano, should never be used in direct contact with your skin. These are best added to a vaporizer or a diffuser for essential oils so that very small amounts are inhaled. Please keep in mind that some essential oils are very toxic to most animals, especially cats. Be mindful of that and keep it out of reach of your pets.

Flower Essence Blends

While the main focus of herbal medicine is on the physical health of the human body, flower essences subtly work to balance our emotional layers. Experiencing extreme emotions such as anger, fear, or grief can stop us from making healthy decisions and can also have a negative effect on us on a physical level. When you choose to work on your emotions with the help of flower essences, it could lead to overall health.

You can put a custom blend together to help you with the mental and emotional challenges that you are facing at any given time. Specific flower essences work well with particular emotions or blockage patterns, discovered through research and study. The Flower Essence Society in California has been conducting this research since 1979. That organization offers endless resources as well as classes and certifications if you would like to learn more.

Fomentations

A fomentation is a very strong herbal brew that is similar to a wash. It is applied by soaking a cotton cloth or cotton in it and placing it on or wrapping it securely around the affected area. Sometimes heat is used to help drive the herbs into the skin. Fomentations are great for applying to your body parts that have no movement or are not able to be lowered in a sitz bath or wash.

One of the favorite uses for fomentations is after any type of body treatment, whether it is massage, acupuncture, or just an adjustment. Ending the body treatment by placing a warm fomentation on the area worked on really helps. The combination of herbs gives off a pleasant aroma that oftentimes evokes healing as it creates a sense of calm relaxation and closure at the end of a treatment. For strains and sprains, this is excellent to use for a first-line treatment. Areas such as your knees and elbows are difficult to soak, so they are perfect candidates for the fomentations. Simply making a lavender and black cohosh fermentation and applying it to the nape of your neck can really do wonders for stress and headaches.

Liniments

Liniments are known as topical applications that can increase your blood circulation and promote healing. Applying liniment on unbroken skin is helpful for sore muscles, aches, and pains. Liniments differ from fomentations because the solution is made with a solvent such as isopropyl alcohol, vinegar, or witch hazel. Liniments have the ability to penetrate and evaporate on your skin surface quickly, but the actions can have lasting effects.

Herbal Oils

Herbal oils are not to be confused with essential oils. Just to be clear, an herbal oil is an herb-infused oil, most often with olive oil, that could be used topically in that form or as a base of another herbal formula such as a lotion, salve, or cream. An essential oil is a distilled product. Both are great and have awesome healing properties, but they are very different from each other.

Medicinal Teas

Herbal teas are the unsung herbal heroes that are able to create significant physiological changes in your body. Most people associate herbal teas with specific flavors rather than with specific medicinal effects. Something considered as insignificant and benign as chamomile tea can have very significant effects on your body. There are women who regularly drink chamomile tea to decrease menstrual cramping and regulate their cycles. Some people like to drink peppermint tea after they have had dinner because they enjoy the taste and want to cleanse their palate. They may not even know that it also helps with your digestion support. Medicinal teas that are made from herbal blends are usually brewed by the cup as needed or in batches designed to provide one day's worth of medicine. It is not recommended to make herbal tea in larger batches because most of the herbs don't keep well after several days. Even while being stored in the refrigerator, some of the herbs, like marshmallow root or slippery elm bark, will make the tea sour and impart a bitter flavor. A batch is usually considered one quart or roughly three 10-ounce cups of the tea. You can make a quart of tea one of two ways; both are equally fine.

Poultices

A poultice has been considered one of the most primitive but very effective ways to use herbs for healing. By definition, a poultice is a damp, soft mass of material, mostly plant material, or plant material mixed with flour. It is applied to the body to relieve soreness and inflammation. The application is in a thick layer, and it is kept in place with a cloth. Some people recommend the use of heat, but it is not always necessary in order for the poultice to be effective. Most of the time your own body heat is effective enough. You may have seen older people cook onions and ginger together when someone had a cold. This was not to eat, but it was mixed with flour and stuffed in an old sock and applied to the throat and neck area. Even though the mixture sounded gross, it really worked to help put you to sleep and reduce the severity of the cold. Taking an herb and mixing it with a little bit of hot water to open it up and placing it on the affected area is the easiest way for you to experience the benefits of natural remedies.

Salves

A salve which is most often applied topically to your skin, is sometime referred to as a balm, ointment, and emollient, or a cream. The base is typically made with beeswax although some people started switching to vegan options such as candelilla wax and Shea butter. When you infuse the herbs into an oil and then add the wax you get a semi-solid substance that can be spread onto the skin wherever it is needed. Back in the day Sal's had basis of bear grease, lard, and whatever other animal fat that they could use.

The salve is used to soothe the body. When you apply a bit of the salve onto whatever is ailing you, it is the easiest way to get the herbs into your skin. Even though you will eventually heal from small cuts, burns, or bug bites, it still feels good to have a touch of relief in the meanwhile. Salves are also great to relieve muscle tension. You can decide whether you want the salve to be scented or not. When you add essential oils to the salve, you want to make sure that it smells good and also adds extra healing potential. When you were using a salve, you didn't need a lot. You always want to cover the area that you have applied the salve to completely. When you have a little bit of salve sitting on top of the injured area, it acts as a natural bandage.

Herbal Spray

Herbal sprays have been widely used over the years, and they are easy to create. You only need a spritz of it here and there, and it could quickly calm inflammation, soothe a cut, shift your emotions, or transfer the smell of a room. Make sure that the sprays you combine are not toxic combinations that irritate your nasal passages.

Herbal Syrups

The base of an herbal syrup is usually a strong herbal tea that has been simmered down and reduced to create a super potent concentrated brew. It is often combined with honey or sugar to create an herbal syrup. This is just another example of how easy it is to make herbal medications. A lot of us are familiar with the elderberry syrup. It is high in antioxidants, and it has antiviral properties. Elderberry is a great addition to any household medicine cabinet. Of course, most of us as children and adults have used cough syrup at some point in our lives. We now know that syrups are not just for flu and colds. Did you know that you can also make a syrup for headaches, to replenish minerals, to make a hair tonic, and to soothe a child's tummy?

Tinctures

Tinctures are created by soaking an herb in alcohol to extract the healing properties from it. This method results in a medicine that can be taken by mouth. Even though temperatures can be made in other ways other than alcohol, such as vinegar or vegetable glycerin, alcohol is the most commonly used form. The advantage of using alcohol is that it works with almost any plant; you can actually formulate the optimal alcohol percentage that a plant's constituents extract, and alcohol-based allows for sublingual transmission. This means that the medicine will bypass the digestive system and go directly into the bloodstream. That is extremely helpful when medicine is needed to treat an acute situation. Some women, while having menstrual cramps, use a tincture because it begins to work right away instead of them taking a capsule and having to wait 40 minutes or so for it to work. I will admit teachers definitely have a strong alcohol flavor, so if you cannot handle that, you should refer to using herbs that can be extracted with apple cider vinegar or vegetable glycerin.

3

Capsules

Many people prefer making their own herbal capsules because it allows for complete control over the ingredients, ensuring purity, quality, and customization to suit individual needs. By crafting their capsules, they can avoid fillers, additives, and synthetic substances often found in commercial products. It also empowers them to tailor blends for specific health goals, such as immune support, stress relief, or digestion, using fresh, trusted herbs. Additionally, DIY capsules are often more cost-effective and offer a hands-on way to connect with natural wellness practices.

Immune-Boosting Herbal Capsules

Support your immune system naturally with this blend of powerful herbs.

Ingredients:

- 2 tablespoons echinacea (dried and powdered)
- 2 tablespoons elderberry (dried and powdered)
- 2 tablespoons turmeric (dried and powdered)
- 1 teaspoon black pepper (dried and powdered, to enhance turmeric absorption)
- Empty size 00 capsules

Instructions:

1. In a small bowl, mix the echinacea, elderberry, turmeric, and black pepper until evenly blended.
2. Using a capsule filler or manually, fill the empty capsules with the herbal mixture.
3. Store the filled capsules in an airtight jar in a cool, dark place.
4. Dosage: Take 1-2 capsules daily with water, especially during cold and flu season.

Digestive Support Herbal Capsules

Soothe your digestive system with this gentle and effective herbal remedy.

Ingredients:

- 2 tablespoons peppermint (dried and powdered)
- 2 tablespoons fennel (dried and powdered)
- 2 tablespoons ginger (dried and powdered)
- Empty size 00 capsules

Instructions:

1. Combine peppermint, fennel, and ginger powder in a bowl, and mix thoroughly.
2. Fill each capsule with the mixture using a capsule filler or by hand.
3. Transfer the capsules to a clean, labeled jar with a tight-fitting lid.
4. Dosage: Take one capsule 30 minutes before meals to promote digestion and to ease bloating.

Stress Relief Herbal Capsules

Promote relaxation and reduce stress with this calming blend.

Ingredients:

- 2 tablespoons ashwagandha (dried and powdered)

- 2 tablespoons lemon balm (dried and powdered)
- 2 tablespoons passionflower (dried and powdered)
- Empty size 00 capsules

Instructions:

1. Mix the ashwagandha, lemon balm, and passionflower powder in a mixing bowl until evenly combined.
2. Use a capsule filler or a small spoon to carefully pack the mixture into empty capsules.
3. Store the capsules in a dry, cool place in a labeled jar.
4. Dosage: Take one capsule in the morning and one capsule at night to promote a sense of calmness.

Each recipe uses natural, powdered herbs and is customizable based on your specific needs. Be sure to consult a healthcare provider before starting new herbal supplements.

4

Essential Oil Blends

Essential oils are popular for their therapeutic properties, offering natural ways to support physical and emotional well-being. They are commonly used in aromatherapy, skincare, and household remedies for stress relief, relaxation, immune support, and more. Their concentrated plant extracts provide potent aromas and benefits, making them versatile for holistic health practices.

Relaxing Lavender Bath Soak

Ingredients:

- 10 drops of lavender essential oil
- 2 cups of Epsom salt
- 1 tablespoon of carrier oil (e.g., coconut or almond oil)

Instructions:

1. Mix the lavender oil with the carrier oil and stir in the Epsom salt.
2. Add the mixture to warm bath water and soak for 20–30 minutes to promote relaxation and better sleep.

Immune-Boosting Roller Blend

Ingredients:

- 5 drops of tea tree essential oil
- 5 drops of eucalyptus essential oil
- 10 ml of carrier oil (e.g., jojoba oil)
- Roller bottle

Instructions:

1. Combine the essential oils with the carrier oil in a roller bottle.
2. Apply to the wrists, neck, or soles of the feet during cold and flu season to support immunity.

Uplifting Citrus Room Spray

Ingredients:

- 10 drops of orange essential oil
- 5 drops of lemon essential oil
- 1 tablespoon of witch hazel
- 1 cup of distilled water
- Spray bottle

Instructions:

1. Mix the essential oils with witch hazel or vodka in a spray bottle.
2. Add the distilled water, shake well, and spritz around your space to create an energizing and fresh atmosphere.

5

Flower Essence Blends

Flower essence blends are gentle remedies made from the energy of flowers. They support emotional balance and well-being, helping with stress, fear, or sadness. Blends combine different essences to enhance their calming and healing effects, offering natural support for the mind and spirit.

Calming Flower Essence Tea

Ingredients:

- 1 cup hot water
- 1 tsp dried chamomile flowers
- 1 tsp dried lavender flowers
- 2 drops Rescue Remedy (Bach Flower Essence blend)

Instructions:

1. Steep chamomile and lavender in hot water for 5-7 minutes.
2. Strain the tea into a cup.
3. Add 2 drops of Rescue Remedy and stir gently.
4. Sip slowly in a peaceful environment.

Healing Benefits:

- **Chamomile** promotes relaxation and reduces stress.

- **Lavender** supports emotional balance and calmness.
- **Rescue Remedy** is a blend of Bach Flower Essences that helps alleviate immediate stress and bring a sense of stability and calm.

Heart-Healing Flower Essence Elixir

Ingredients:

- 1 cup filtered water
- 1 tsp rose petals (fresh or dried)
- 1 tsp hibiscus petals
- 2 drops rose flower essence blend (for emotional healing and self-love)

Instructions:

1. Combine rose and hibiscus petals with water in a saucepan.
2. Gently heat to a simmer for 5 minutes, then strain.
3. Add 2 drops of rose flower essence blend.
4. Drink warm or cool as desired.

Healing Benefits:

- **Rose petals** open the heart, fostering love and compassion.
- **Hibiscus** enhances feelings of joy and vitality.
- **Rose flower essence** helps release emotional pain and cultivate self-acceptance and inner peace.

Energy Renewal Mist

Ingredients:

- 1 small spray bottle
- 1 cup distilled water
- 3 drops orange blossom essence (for vitality)
- 2 drops yarrow flower essence (for energetic protection)
- Optional: 1 drop of essential oil (e.g., peppermint for energy boost)

Instructions:

1. Fill the spray bottle with distilled water.
2. Add the flower essences and essential oil.
3. Shake well before each use.
4. Spray around yourself or in your space for an energy refresh.

Healing Benefits:

- **Orange blossom essence** revitalizes energy and inspires creativity.
- **Yarrow essence** creates a protective energetic shield, enhancing focus.
- **Peppermint essential oil** invigorates and clears mental fog.

Each recipe is a gentle way to incorporate the healing vibrations of flowers, working on emotional, mental, and spiritual levels.

6

Fomentations

Fomentations are warm or cold compresses applied to the body to soothe pain, reduce inflammation, or improve circulation. They're often made by soaking cloths in herbal infusions or essential oil solutions and placing them on the affected area. Whether for relaxation, healing, or comfort, fomentations are a simple, natural remedy.

Chamomile Relaxation Compress

Ingredients:

- 2 cups boiling water
- 2 tablespoons dried chamomile flowers
- 1 clean cloth.

Instructions:

Steep chamomile flowers in boiling water for 10 minutes. Strain, soak the cloth in the liquid, wring out excess, and apply warm to the desired area.

Ginger & Turmeric Soothe Compress

Ingredients:

- 2 cups boiling water
- 1 tablespoon grated ginger
- 1 teaspoon turmeric powder
- 1 clean cloth.

Instructions:

Simmer ginger and turmeric in water for 5 minutes. Strain, soak the cloth, wring it out, and apply warmth to ease soreness.

Peppermint Cooling Compress

Ingredients:

- 2 cups cool water
- 5 drops peppermint essential oil
- 1 clean cloth.

Instructions:

Mix peppermint oil into cool water. Soak the cloth, wring it out, and apply it to areas needing cooling relief.

7

Liniments

Liniments are liquid herbal remedies applied to the skin to relieve aches, pains, or stiffness. They're typically made with a base of alcohol or oil infused with healing herbs or essential oils. Liniments are easy to use and can provide quick relief when massaged onto sore areas.

Arnica Muscle-Soothing Liniment

Ingredients:

- 1 cup rubbing alcohol
- 2 tablespoons dried arnica flowers
- 10 drops eucalyptus essential oil.

Instructions:

Combine arnica flowers and alcohol in a jar and let it sit for two weeks, shaking daily. Strain, add eucalyptus oil, and store in a bottle. Apply to sore muscles as needed.

Cayenne Warming Liniment

Ingredients:

- 1 cup olive oil
- 1 tablespoon cayenne pepper

- 1 teaspoon ginger powder.

Instructions:

Heat the oil gently and stir in cayenne and ginger. Let it cool, strain, and store in a bottle. Massage onto stiff joints or cold hands and feet.

Lavender Relaxation Liniment

Ingredients:

- 1 cup witch hazel
- 10 drops lavender essential oil
- 1 teaspoon dried lavender buds.

Instructions:

Mix lavender buds and witch hazel in a jar. Infuse for one week, strain, and add essential oil. Massage onto the skin for calming relief.

8

Herbal Oils

Herbal oils are made by infusing herbs into a carrier oil to capture their therapeutic properties. They're used for massages, skincare, or healing minor ailments like dry skin, soreness, or irritation. These oils are versatile and easy to make at home.

Calendula Healing Oil

Ingredients:

- 1 cup olive oil
- ½ cup dried calendula flowers.

Instructions:

Place calendula flowers in a clean jar and cover with olive oil. Seal the jar and let it infuse in a warm spot for four weeks, shaking occasionally. Strain and store in a dark bottle. Use for dry or irritated skin.

Rosemary Hair-Nourishing Oil

Ingredients:

- 1 cup coconut oil
- ¼ cup fresh rosemary sprigs.

Instructions:

Gently heat coconut oil and rosemary in a saucepan for 20 minutes. Cool, strain, and store in a jar. Massage into your scalp to promote healthy hair growth.

Lavender Relaxation Oil

Ingredients:

- 1 cup almond oil
- 2 tablespoons dried lavender buds
- 10 drops lavender essential oil.

Instructions:

1. Combine lavender buds and almond oil in a jar.
2. Let it infuse for three weeks, shaking occasionally.
3. Strain, add lavender essential oil, and store in a bottle.
4. Use for massages or as a calming body oil.

9

Medicinal Teas

What Are Medicinal Teas?

Medicinal teas are herbal infusions made to support health and well-being. They combine healing herbs with hot water to create soothing remedies for various ailments, from colds to stress. Easy to prepare, they are a natural way to care for your body and mind.

Immune-Boosting Elderberry Tea

Ingredients:

- 2 cups boiling water
- 1 tablespoon dried elderberries
- 1 teaspoon dried echinacea
- 1 teaspoon honey (optional).

Instructions:

1. Combine elderberries and echinacea in a teapot, pour in boiling water, and steep for 10 minutes.
2. Strain, sweeten with honey if desired, and enjoy.

Calming Chamomile & Lemon Balm Tea

Ingredients:

- 1 cup boiling water
- 1 teaspoon dried chamomile flowers
- 1 teaspoon dried lemon balm leaves.

Instructions:

1. Add chamomile and lemon balm to a cup, pour in boiling water, and steep for 5-7 minutes.
2. Strain and drink to ease stress or aid sleep.

Digestive Ginger & Peppermint Tea

Ingredients:

- 1 cup boiling water
- 1 teaspoon fresh grated ginger
- 1 teaspoon dried peppermint leaves.

Instructions:

1. Place ginger and peppermint in a mug, pour in boiling water, and steep for 10 minutes.
2. Strain and sip slowly to soothe digestion.

10

Poultices

Poultices are soft, moist herbal mixtures applied directly to the skin to reduce swelling, soothe pain, or promote healing. They're typically made from fresh or dried herbs and can be used warm or cool, depending on the condition being treated.

Soothing Plantain Poultice

Ingredients:

- ½ cup fresh plantain leaves
- 2 tablespoons warm water
- clean cloth or bandage.

Instructions:

1. Mash plantain leaves with warm water to form a paste.
2. Spread the mixture on a cloth and apply it to cuts, bites, or rashes. Secure with a bandage and leave for 20-30 minutes.

Anti-Inflammatory Turmeric Poultice

Ingredients:

- 1 tablespoon turmeric powder
- 1 tablespoon flour

- 2 tablespoons warm water
- clean cloth.

Instructions:

1. Mix turmeric, flour, and warm water into a thick paste.
2. Spread it on the cloth and place it on the affected area.
3. Leave for 15-20 minutes to reduce swelling or pain.

Cooling Cabbage Poultice

Ingredients:

- 2-3 large cabbage leaves
- warm water
- clean cloth, or bandage.

Instructions:

1. Soften cabbage leaves by dipping them in warm water.
2. Lay the leaves directly on swollen or painful areas, secure with a bandage, and leave for 30-60 minutes.

11

Salves

Salves are semi-solid ointments or balms made from oils, waxes, and medicinal herbs. They are commonly used in natural and herbal medicine to soothe, protect, or treat various skin conditions and other external ailments.

Salves are easy to apply, remain on the surface of the skin, and provide a localized effect rather than being absorbed systemically.Salves are an integral part of herbal medicine, and most people like them because of how easy it is to apply, their effectiveness, and the ability to customize them to specific needs by varying the herbs used in their preparation.

Healing Lavender and Calendula Salve

Perfect for soothing burns, cuts, and dry skin.

Ingredients:

- 1 cup olive oil (infused with dried lavender and calendula flowers)
- 1 ounce beeswax (grated or pellets)
- 10 drops of lavender essential oil
- 5 drops of tea tree essential oil
- 1 teaspoon vitamin E oil (optional, for preservation)

Instructions:

Infuse the Oil

1. Combine ½ cup dried lavender flowers and ½ cup dried calendula flowers with 1 cup olive oil in a double boiler or slow cooker.
2. Heat on low for 2-3 hours, ensuring the oil does not overheat or burn. Strain through cheesecloth into a clean glass jar.

Prepare the Salve

3. In a double boiler, melt the beeswax over low heat.
4. Add the infused oil and stir until fully combined.
5. Add Essential Oils
6. Remove the mixture from heat and stir in lavender, tea tree essential oils, and vitamin E oil.

Pour and Set

7. Pour the mixture into sterilized tins or jars. Let it cool completely before sealing.

Peppermint and Eucalyptus Muscle-Relief Salve

Relieves sore muscles and minor aches.

Ingredients:

- 1 cup coconut oil
- 1 ounce beeswax (grated or pellets)
- 15 drops peppermint essential oil
- 10 drops eucalyptus essential oil
- 10 drops of arnica
- 5 drops of rosemary essential oil
- 1 teaspoon menthol crystals (optional, for extra cooling effect)

Instructions:

Melt the Base Ingredients

1. In a double boiler, melt the coconut oil and beeswax over low heat.
2. Stir until the mixture is fully liquified.

Incorporate Essential Oils

3. Remove from heat and add the peppermint, eucalyptus, and rosemary essential oils. If using menthol crystals, stir them in while the mixture is warm to dissolve.

Pour and Cool

4. Pour the mixture into tins or jars. Allow it to solidify at room temperature.

Label and Store

5. Label the jars and store them in a cool, dry place.

Antiseptic Thyme and Chamomile Salve

Great for minor cuts, insect bites, and irritations.

Ingredients:

- 1 cup sweet almond oil (infused with dried thyme and chamomile)
- 1 ounce beeswax (grated or pellets)
- 10 drops of chamomile essential oil
- 10 drops of frankincense essential oil
- 1 teaspoon honey (optional, for additional healing properties)

Instructions:

Create the Infused Oil

1. Combine ½ cup dried thyme and ½ cup dried chamomile with the almond oil in a heat-proof jar.
2. Place the jar in a water bath and simmer on low heat for 2-3 hours. Strain the oil into a clean container.

Melt and Combine

3. In a double boiler, melt the beeswax. Add the infused oil and stir until well blended.

Add the Finishing Touches

4. Stir in chamomile and frankincense essential oils. If using honey, add it now and mix thoroughly.

Pour and Let Set

5. Transfer the mixture to sterilized tins or jars. Let it cool and

solidify completely.

Keep This In Mind For All Recipes:

6. Storage: Keep salves in a cool, dark place. They typically last 6-12 months with proper storage.
7. Customization: Adjust essential oils to suit your preferences or skin sensitivities.
8. Safety: Test a small amount on your skin before full use to ensure no allergic reactions.

12

Herbal Sprays

Herbal sprays are liquid remedies made from herbal infusions, essential oils, or tinctures, used for refreshing, cleansing, or healing. They're versatile and easy to make, perfect for skincare, room freshening, or addressing minor ailments like bug bites or dry skin.

Lavender Sleep Spray

Ingredients:

- 1 cup distilled water
- 10 drops lavender essential oil
- 1 teaspoon witch hazel.

Instructions:

Combine all ingredients in a spray bottle and shake well. Mist pillows or linens before bed to promote relaxation and restful sleep.

Cooling Aloe & Peppermint Spray

Ingredients:

- ½ cup aloe vera juice
- ½ cup distilled water

- 5 drops peppermint essential oil.

Instructions:

1. Mix all ingredients in a spray bottle and shake.
2. Spray onto sunburns or hot skin for soothing, cooling relief.

Anti-Bug Herbal Spray

Ingredients:

- 1 cup distilled water
- 1 tablespoon dried rosemary
- 1 tablespoon dried thyme
- 10 drops citronella essential oil.

Instructions:

1. Boil water, steep rosemary and thyme for 20 minutes, then strain.
2. Let cool, add citronella oil, and pour into a spray bottle.
3. Use to repel insects naturally.

13

Herbal Syrups

Herbal syrups are sweet, thick liquid remedies made by combining herbal infusions or decoctions with sugar or honey. They're a delicious way to deliver the healing properties of herbs, often used to soothe coughs, boost immunity, or support digestion.

Elderberry Immune Syrup

Ingredients:

- 1 cup dried elderberries
- 4 cups water
- 1 cup raw honey.

Instructions:

1. Simmer elderberries in water for 30 minutes. Strain and cool slightly.
2. Stir in honey until dissolved. Store in a sealed jar in the refrigerator and take 1-2 teaspoons daily for immune support.

Ginger & Thyme Pineapple Cough Syrup

Ingredients:

- ¼ cup fresh ginger slices

- fresh pineapple
- 2 tablespoons dried thyme
- 2 cups water
- 1 cup honey.

Instructions:

1. Simmer ginger, pineapple, and thyme in water for 20 minutes, and strain.
2. Let cool slightly, add honey, and mix well.
3. Store in a jar and take 1 tablespoon as needed for cough relief.

Lemon Balm Calming Syrup

Ingredients:

- 1 cup dried lemon balm
- 2 cups water
- 1 cup sugar.

Instructions:

1. Boil lemon balm in water for 15 minutes, then strain.
2. Stir in sugar while the liquid is warm until fully dissolved.
3. Store in a bottle in the refrigerator and use 1-2 teaspoons to ease stress or anxiety.

14

Tinctures

Tinctures are concentrated herbal extracts made by steeping herbs in alcohol or glycerin. They are powerful and easy to use so that you can enjoy the benefits of the herbs. A few drops of tincture can be taken under the tongue or diluted in water for wellness support.

Echinacea Immune-Boosting Tincture

Ingredients:

- 1 cup dried echinacea root
- 2 cups vodka (80 proof or higher).

Instructions:

1. Place the echinacea in a jar, cover completely with vodka, and seal tightly.
2. Let it steep in a dark place for 4-6 weeks, shaking occasionally. Strain and store in a dropper bottle.
3. Take 1-2 droppers at the first sign of a cold.

Chamomile Calming Tincture

Ingredients:

- 1 cup dried chamomile flowers

- 2 cups brandy.

Instructions:

1. Add chamomile to a jar, pour in brandy to cover completely, and seal. Steep in a cool, dark place for four weeks, shaking daily.
2. Strain and store.
3. Take 1-2 droppers as needed to ease stress or promote sleep.

Peppermint Digestive Tincture

Ingredients:

- 1 cup fresh peppermint leaves,
- 2 cups grain alcohol or vodka.

Instructions:

1. Fill a jar with peppermint leaves and cover with alcohol.
2. Seal and steep for 3-4 weeks in a dark place, shaking regularly.
3. Strain and store.
4. Use 10-15 drops in water to support digestion.

15

Natural Remedies and Practices for Wellness

The Rainbow Diet: Eating for Vibrancy and Health

Incorporate a variety of colorful fruits and vegetables to maximize nutrient intake.

Whenever possible, choose organic or sustainably sourced produce to avoid harmful pesticides.

Buy local: Supporting farmers' markets ensures freshness and sustainability.

Vegetables: Include spinach, kale, bell peppers, and beets for antioxidants and essential vitamins.

Fruits: Add berries, citrus fruits, and apples for immune support and digestion.

Herbal Infusions: Drink nettle or dandelion tea to enhance mineral intake and support liver health.

Spices: Incorporate turmeric (anti-inflammatory), ginger (digestion), and cinnamon (blood sugar regulation).

Fats and Proteins for Optimal Health

Choose healthy fats: avocados, olive oil, coconut oil, nuts, and seeds.

Limit vegetable oils and fried foods, as they can contribute to inflammation.

Prioritize quality proteins: wild-caught fish, pasture-raised poultry, and lean meats.

Healing Fats and Proteins

Use flaxseed oil or chia seeds for omega-3 fatty acids.

Supplement with moringa powder for a plant-based protein boost and essential amino acids.

Foods to Avoid for Better Health

Processed or refined sugars, sodas, and artificial sweeteners.

Bleached grains and overprocessed foods.

Reduce alcohol and caffeine to promote balanced energy levels.

Practical Tips

Stay hydrated: Drink filtered or spring water from stainless steel containers.

Aim for whole grains and natural sweeteners like honey or agave nectar.

Exercise Matters. Movement Is Vitality

Regular exercise, even as simple as walking or stretching, offers numerous benefits:

- Slows the aging process.
- Improves energy levels, mood, and brain function.
- Reduces the risk of heart disease, diabetes, and cancer.

Herbal Aids for Energy and Recovery

Ashwagandha: A powerful adaptogen that reduces stress and improves energy levels.

Ginseng: Enhances physical stamina and mental focus.

Gotu Kola: Supports circulation and promotes recovery after exercise.

Creating a Routine

Pair exercise with an herbal recovery tea like peppermint or chamomile to relax muscles and reduce inflammation.

Start small: Find activities you enjoy and can sustain, such as yoga, dancing, or swimming.Aim for at least 30 minutes of movement five days a week.

Foundational Supplements

Healing with Supplements and Herbal Remedies

Multivitamins: Choose whole-food-based options for better absorption.

Essential Oils: Flax or fish oil provides Omega-3 fatty acids for heart and brain health.

Vitamin D3: Take 1,000–5,000 IU/day to maintain optimal levels.

Vitamin C: Take as much as your digestion tolerates for immune support.

Probiotics: Strengthen gut health and immunity with daily use.

Herbal Allies

Elderberry: A powerful antiviral to boost recovery during illness.

Echinacea: Supports immunity when taken at the first sign of a cold.

Chamomile and Peppermint Teas: Aid digestion and relaxation.

Hibiscus Tea: Helps reduce blood pressure when consumed regularly.

Holy Basil (Tulsi): A natural adaptogen that supports immunity and combats stress.

Milk Thistle: Protects and detoxifies the liver.

Fenugreek: Improves digestion and helps regulate blood sugar.

Signs You Need a Detox

Persistent fatigue, skin rashes, headaches, or digestive discomfort.

Increased sensitivity to allergens or environmental irritants.

Simple Detox Practices

1. **Healthy Eating**: Avoid sugar, alcohol, and processed foods. Focus on vegetables, fruits, and lean proteins.
2. **Juice Fasting**: Incorporate raw vegetable juices like zucchini, beets, carrots, and leafy greens.
3. **Hydration**: Drink plenty of water with fresh lemon juice to support liver health.

Supportive Measures

Skin Brushing: Stimulates lymphatic drainage and detoxifies the skin.

Lymphatic Massage: Helps eliminate toxins stored in tissues.

Colon Hydrotherapy: Use cautiously under professional supervision.

Detox Herbs

Dandelion Root: A gentle liver cleanser that promotes bile flow.

Burdock Root: Supports kidney function and purifies the blood.

Calendula: A mild detoxifier that aids in lymphatic drainage.

Herbal Teas for Detox

Horsetail Tea: Rich in silica, supports skin and hair health.

Peppermint and Licorice Tea: Aids digestion and soothes the stomach.

Ginger and Lemon Tea: Boosts circulation and enhances detoxification.

Daily Habits for Immune Health

Get 8–9 hours of quality sleep in a dark room free of artificial light.

Wash your hands frequently and avoid touching your face unnecessarily.

Limit refined sugar, which suppresses the immune system for hours after consumption.

Daily Herbal Immune Boosters

Elderberry Syrup: Prevents and shortens colds and flu.

Echinacea: Activates white blood cells to fight infections.

Astragalus: A traditional Chinese herb that strengthens long-term immunity.

Natural Remedies During Illness

Vitamin C: Take high doses (as tolerated) to speed recovery.

Zinc: Start with 75–100 mg on the first day, reducing to 30 mg daily until recovery.

Elderberry and Olive Leaf Extract: Use these natural antivirals to shorten illness duration. Fights viral infections and reduces inflammation.

Probiotics: Support your gut's immune system by taking them hourly at the onset of symptoms.

Thyme Tea: Acts as a natural antiseptic for respiratory issues.

Propolis: A resin from bees with potent antiviral and antibacterial properties.

Managing High Blood Pressure Naturally

High blood pressure increases the risk of stroke and heart disease. Symptoms may include headaches, fatigue, or dizziness.

Natural Solutions and Diet Adjustments:

- Increase potassium-rich foods like bananas, avocados, and leafy greens.
- Avoid high-sodium foods like canned goods and chips.
- Include garlic, asparagus, and spices in your meals.

Herbal Remedies:

- **Hibiscus Tea**: Proven to help reduce blood pressure when consumed daily.
- **Pomegranate Juice**: Unsweetened varieties can improve heart health.
- **Garlic**: Take fresh garlic or aged garlic extract for heart health.
- **Valerian Root**: Reduces stress-induced blood pressure spikes.

Lifestyle Tips:

- Limit caffeine and alcohol.
- Incorporate calming practices like meditation or yoga to reduce stress.
- Avoid salty foods and add potassium-rich options like sweet potatoes and spinach.
- Drink beet juice or pomegranate juice daily to support healthy circulation.

Creating a Restful Environment and Sleep Sanctuary

- Darken your room and eliminate artificial light at night.
- Use natural materials in your bedding for better air circulation.
- use lavender essential oil for relaxation.

Herbal Aids for Sleep

- **Chamomile:** Soothes the nervous system and promotes restful sleep.
- **Passionflower**: Reduces anxiety and helps with insomnia.
- **Lemon Balm**: Calms the mind and enhances sleep quality.
- Use **Lavender** essential oil for relaxation.
- Brew a **Valerian Root Tea** or take it as a tincture for deep relaxation before bedtime.

Restorative Sleep Tips

- Sleep 8–9 hours per night to allow your body to heal and recharge.
- Short naps during the day are okay if they don't disrupt nighttime sleep.

Here are some quick herbal remedies for common ailments:

Digestive Issues

- **Peppermint Tea**: Relieves bloating and gas.
- **Slippery Elm Bark**: Soothes digestive tract lining.
- **Fennel Seeds**: Chew after meals for improved digestion.
- **Chamomile**: Reduces nausea and calms the stomach.
- **Ginger**: Aids digestion, reduces nausea, and prevents bloating.
- **Licorice Root**: Soothes heartburn and gastric discomfort.
- **Dandelion Root Tea**: Supports liver health and stimulates digestion.
- **Caraway Seeds**: Relieve bloating, gas, and indigestion.
- **Cinnamon**:Promotes digestion and reduces stomach cramps.

Headaches

- **Feverfew**: Prevents migraines and reduces their intensity.
- **Willow Bark**: A natural alternative to aspirin.
- **Lavender**: Aromatherapy or tea reduces tension headaches.
- **Peppermint Oil**:Applied topically to relieve tension headaches.
- **Butterbur**: Reduces frequency and severity of migraines.
- **Rosemary Tea**: Improves circulation and reduces headache pain.
- **GingerTea**: Reduces headache symptoms caused by inflammation.
- **Valerian Root**: Soothes tension headaches and promotes relaxation.

Skin Health

- **Aloe Vera Gel**: Soothes burns and promote healing.
- **Neem Oil**: Treats acne and skin infections.
- **Calendula**: Promoteshealingofwoundsandreducesinflammation.
- **Tea Tree Oil**: Antimicrobial properties for acne and fungal infections.

- **Witch Hazel**: Soothes skin irritation and reduces swelling.
- **Burdock Root**: Detoxifies the skin and clears eczema.
- **Horsetail**: Strengthens skin, hair, and nails with its silica content.
- **Gotu Kola**: Promotes wound healing and improves skin elasticity.
- **Comfrey**: Speeds healing of wounds, bruises, and burns.
- **Chickweed**: Soothes itchy and irritated skin.

Joint Pain

- **Turmeric& Black Pepper**: Anti-inflammatoryand pain-relieving properties.
- **Boswellia (Frankincense)**: Reduces inflammation in arthritis.
- **Devil's Claw**: Effective for joint and back pain.
- **Ginger**: Reduces inflammation and alleviates stiffness.
- **Nettle Leaf Tea**: Eases joint inflammation and supports bone health.
- **Eucalyptus Oil**: Applied topically to soothe joint pain.
- **Ashwagandha**: Reduces inflammation and improves mobility.
- **Cat's Claw**: Alleviates joint pain by reducing inflammation.

Women's Health Issues

Menstrual Health

- **Raspberry Leaf Tea**: Regulates menstrual cycles and relieves cramps.
- **Cramp Bark**: Reduces uterine cramps and discomfort.
- **Ginger Tea**: Eases menstrual pain and reduces inflammation.
- **Dong Quai**: Balances hormones and improves circulation to the uterus.
- **Chamomile**: Calms PMS symptoms and reduces pain.

Hormonal Balance

- **Vitex (Chasteberry)**: Regulates menstrual cycles and reduces PMS symptoms.
- **Ashwagandha**: Reduces stress and supports adrenal health.
- **Maca Root**: Balances hormones and boosts energy.

- **Black Cohosh**: Eases menopause symptoms like hot flashes.
- **Evening Primrose Oil**: Helpswithhormonalacneandbreast tenderness.

Reproductive Health

- **Red Clover**: Supports fertility by balancing hormones.
- **Shatavari**: A traditional Ayurvedic herb for female reproductive health.
- **Nettle Leaf**: Nourishes the uterus and boosts iron levels.
- **Lady'sMantle**: Strengthens the uterine lining and regulates cycles.

Urinary Health

- **Cranberry**: Prevents and treats urinary tract infections (UTIs).
- **Uva Ursi (Bearberry)**: Soothes urinary tract infections.
- **Parsley Tea**: Acts as a mild diuretic to support urinary health.

Lactation Support

- **Fenugreek**: Enhances milk production.
- **Milk Thistle**: Supports lactation and liver health.
- **Blessed Thistle**: Boosts milk supply and supports postpartum recovery.

Menopause

- **Black Cohosh**: Reduces hot flashes and mood swings.
- **Sage**: Relieves night sweats and hot flashes.
- **Licorice Root**: Balances hormones and supports adrenal function.
- **Hops**: Eases insomnia and irritability.

16

Testimonials

Disclaimer: I am not a doctor, and I do not make medical claims.

I am an herbalist that makes miracle claims.

"I can't thank Miss Cotton enough for creating such amazing products! A few years ago, I had a botched wig install and removal that left my scalp in terrible shape. My dermatitis was scratched up so badly that I had scabs everywhere and my edges completely came out, and both of my eyes were infected. I was devastated. After using Miss Cotton's products (shampoo, hair grease, and conditioner), my scalp healed beautifully, and my edges grew back in full! I'm beyond grateful for the care and thought she puts into her products—they truly work wonders. Thank you, Miss Cotton, for helping me restore my confidence!"

- Felicia Cook

I don't know where to begin to say how grateful and appreciative I am that divine planning had Yolanda MissCotton Justice, the healer, come along on my journey. Her healing hands have cared for my crown of glory with her herbs and her hair products. I fell in love with her soaps. I have always gotten compliments on how glowing my skin is. Her teas and capsules of either overall or something specific are nothing but a masterpiece of good health; she has made personal teas or capsules just for me, and I feel great and healed after not just taking them but putting in the work to activate, with gratitude to my ancestors and Creator. I don't have high blood pressure, diabetes, or any major health issues in my lifestyle of herbs thanks to Yolanda MissCotton Justice.

- Conwaja Brunson-Brice

Custom Cancer Fighting Tea and Capsules - special anointed mix, milk thistle, peppermint, ashwagandha, curcumin mistletoe, dandelion root, mullein, cardamom pod, black peppercorn, cinnamon bark, burdock root, fennel seed, clove bud, juniper berry, licorice root, orange peel, pau d' arco bark, sassafras root bark, ginger root, uva ursi leaf, horsetail herb, dandelion leaf, parsley leaf, turmeric powder.

This tea is the ultimate healer of the organs and digestive system. It soothes any gut issues and repairs the damage done to the esophagus and digestive tract. It also helps with nausea, narcotic withdrawal relief, nicotine withdrawal relief, and chemotherapy sickness relief. Thank you, Sis!

-T.C.

Praise Update!

T.C. had his tumor removed, and when they looked at it, *all of the cells were dead!*

The whole time his doctors have been amazed at how well he has done. I know that it was the prayer, and the herbs prayed over and prepared! T.C. only has to return for scans in October and three months after that! And you know when the tumors are removed, the cells are usually still alive—ready to knuck if you buck, as soon as they stop chemo!

We Red Tea—

Mullein, hibiscus, beet root powder, celery powder, turmeric, dandelion root (roasted), cardamom pod, black peppercorn, cinnamon bark, burdock root, clove bud, juniper berry, licorice root, orange peel, pau d' arco bark, sassafras root bark, ginger root, uva ursi leaf.

Anti-inflammatory benefits. Weight loss aid. Improves digestive tract issues. Helps balance blood sugar. Improves insulin resistance in the body. It relieves high blood pressure. Supports a healthy head of hair.

I ordered this tea for my mother-in-law because she was having issues with her blood pressure. After she finished what I ordered, she had me order more for her because she started seeing a positive change. Now I've started drinking it as a precautionary since high blood pressure runs in my family. Awesome product!

- Vellenise G.

I ordered this tea because I was tired of taking blood pressure medicine. I've been on different meds for over 10 years. I started drinking this tea a little over a week ago, and here are my observations: I used to take a blood pressure pill twice a day and a diuretic—this tea is a natural diuretic! I no longer have double vision (which I believe was caused by the BP pills). I feel better overall in my body. I'm excited about the progress so far, and I can't wait to go back to the doctor for my BP check in a couple of months.

- Avery

I purchased this product for my sister; after only three days, she went to her doctor's appointment, and he asked her what she was doing differently. Her numbers are beginning to level off. Thank you so much! I absolutely love this product!

- Tyneka R.

I take We Red Tea Capsules, so this was my first time trying the product. I felt it working with just a few sips along with the capsules, and I've been super calm throughout the day. Dr. Feel Good in tea form. Definitely a must-have.

- Aurelia M.

NoMo Blues Tea—

Mullein, hibiscus, strawberry leaf, gotu kola, ashwagandha, ginseng, ginkgo, red clover, rooibos, echinacea, lemongrass, elderberry, butterfly pea flower.

Improves mood, eyesight, focus, energy, hair growth, and glowing skin.

Aphrodisiac, antioxidant, anti-aging. It can help reduce fatigue and bring about a sense of calm due to the herb's anti-inflammatory and analgesic properties.

It has some stress-busting effects that will also help reduce symptoms of anxiety. Great natural way to refresh the brain and helps keep you energized and happy throughout the day.

This tea is delicious, y'all lol! I can tell the difference after drinking it; I don't have "brain fog" anymore, my appetite has decreased, and I have more energy, and I am more productive at work. I can't wait to place another order!

- Tisha

This is one of my favorites! My skin has never glowed the way it does now since I've been drinking this tea, and I feel youthful looking. People around me recognize it as well, even though they think it's a man. It definitely has improved my eyesight, more focused, and a big burst of energy in an 8 oz cup. You can't beat that!

- Aurelia M.

This tea provides an instant calming effect and an overall feeling of peace. If you have a lot on your mind or want to improve your mood, give this tea a try.

- Denise A.

This is Adderall in a cup. It mellows you out and lifts your mood. That's good; let's get some things done type of mood. I drink this tea once a day to get my day in motion.

- Porchia

Claritea

Mullein, eucalyptus, oregano, peppermint, lobelia, chaparral, elecampane, lungwort, plantain leaf, osha root, skullcap, and Cordyceps, rose hips, rose petals, ginger, anise seed, thyme, yarrow, calendula, and lavender.

Allergy relief, flu relief, lung repair for any lung issues, removal of mucus buildup, calming anxiety, an overall sense of well-being, and boosting the immune system naturally. This was the tea of choice at the height of the COVID-19 pandemic. No caffeine. It really helps to hold your face over the steam to open nasal passages.

I have sinus issues (my husband also sleeps with a fan on), so I have year-round congestion. I bought this tea, and let me tell you… The next thing I knew, the mucus in my chest was gone. All of the teas are good, but this one right here is my favorite!

-Tamicka W.

I'd been trying to get rid of chest congestion for over two months now. I took every name brand over-the-counter decongestant I could find and mixed everything in my green tea, but the kitchen sink and nothing worked. I started drinking the Claritea two days ago, and for the first time I'm not wheezing and don't hear the likes of a fireplace fire crackling in my chest. I'm also sleeping like a baby! You have a customer for life!

-Raechell P.

The name speaks for itself because it literally brought CLAR-ITY to my life!

I wasn't a huge tea drinker until running into Auntie Cotton (in my head) teas, and man, am I grateful. When someone makes something with love and proper intentions, it shows through its customers, like myself, actually writing a REAL LIVE review!

I can't wait to see her products in stores WORLDWIDE. I would say nationwide, but my brain is too big for that small stuff!

-Deedee

Let me please take a moment to express how this tea has changed my symptoms while currently dealing with COVID 19. I tested positive for the virus back on 12/24/2024. Since then, I had been dealing with fevers and chills, confusion, headaches, body aches, cough congestion, fatigue, and most importantly, shortness of breath. I had been going back and forth to emergency rooms for everything and given so much medicine.

Due to the high levels of COVID patients in the hospitals, the doctors told me that my oxygen levels were not low enough to be on a ventilator; all they could do was provide me with a pump and give me oxygen while I was there (like they know how I feel).

My dear friend at work had been keeping up with me and knew that I was not getting any better. I was at the point of believing I was not going to make it. She brought me the ClariTea along with some sea moss and instructed me on how to properly use it.

My God—within 24 hours—my headache, body aches, fatigue, confusion, clouded mind, chills, and cough were all under control. This was a blessing to me. COVID is nothing to play with. This virus has taken everything out of me, and to finally have a day of peace and feel like myself is everything to me. I was in tears because I knew I was going to be okay.

I just want to say thank you and spread my testimony because this was my life on the line and how precious life is.

Thank you to my friend, Lady D, for bringing this to me because, God as my witness, IT WORKS AND I WANT MORE :), GOD BLESS.

-Natosha L.

Oh Baby Fertilitea

***Due to pending patents, the complete formula cannot be disclosed.**

Mullein, an anointed fertility blend, maca root, horny goat weed, red ginseng, organic cinnamon, organic damiana, organic ashwagandha root, organic nettle leaf, organic rose petals.

This special Auntea Baby mix has been proven to produce many pregnancies that can be confirmed. At least 40, including Miss Cotton's own grandbabies!

It balances hormones and ovulation to allow pregnancy. Heals the womb from issues blocking pregnancy, including PCOS and fibroids.

Blessings!

What do you want to be when you grow up? Some children say firefighter, some say teacher, but not me. From a child, I had a dream of being a mother. I knew I would grow up and have children. So, imagine how devastating it was when I thought that would never happen. In 2019 my husband and I discovered we were pregnant. We were so elated; however, the excitement was short-lived when we lost the baby at only 10 weeks. A short year later we dealt with another loss.

Some doctors, family, and friends all gave up on us having a child together. I was told to be grateful that God had blessed me to be able to adopt an amazing son. I was also told that because my husband already had a son, it shouldn't matter anyway. That was not my desire. Miss Cotton stepped in and told me that she had something for me. She told me I needed to heal my womb and that I *would* have a healthy baby. She provided me with herbs that she had blended and prayed over and then prayed over me. One year later we found out we were now in our 3rd pregnancy. I informed her, and she immediately began to pray over me. My son came out healthy and stronger than me! We now have a 3-year-old no-limit soldier.

Also, during COVID, my husband worked at the county hospital. When he caught COVID, Miss Cotton provided us with an herbal blend that not only limited the symptoms my husband had, but I also felt safe giving it to my infant son. My household was protected. I have not only experienced the work of Miss Cotton; I have also heard other stories of those she has helped.

-Avie Mac

I was planning in vitro fertilization and started drinking this tea. I got pregnant and carried 40 weeks to deliver a 9-pound baby! No physician needed!

-Tori B.

I was recently diagnosed a year ago with Polycystic Syndrome, also known as PCOS. It has been a very hard process to have normal monthly cycles, as well as to conceive. My husband and I have experienced three miscarriages. One was due to trauma from a very bad wreck that I was in that shattered my hips and broke my pelvic bone. The other two were unknown of the cause. I conceived last year by using a fertility medicine called Clomid, but that pregnancy ended in one of the miscarriages. I was also put on the medicine Metformin to regulate ovulation, but it still wasn't working. I was very torn and didn't have any more hope left until one day I learned about this awesome Fertilitea. I was so afraid to try it because I didn't want to get my hopes up. However, I made my purchase, and upon picking up my product, Mrs. Justice warned me to only take this tea if I wanted to become pregnant.

The confidence she had in her product was wonderful, but the confidence that she had in her prayers behind the product won me over! I drank two full gallons of the Fertilitea starting on Father's Day 2020 and found out that I was pregnant in July of 2020. I am so very proud to announce that my husband and I are expecting our son in March of 2021.

I know that God used Mrs. Justice and this Fertilitea to bless our family. I couldn't be any more grateful! I continue to help those who have experienced the things I've gone through, and I highly recommend this tea to every woman who is trying to have a baby. No matter what the doctors say, God has the final say. Before you give up, please try this Fertilitea!

Na'koia

I suffer from endometriosis and struggled to get pregnant with my second child. The doctor put me on several rounds of Clomid to help me Super Ovulate, but it didn't work. He wanted me to do another round, but this time I started drinking the FertiliTea with the Clomid. Two weeks later, I found out I was pregnant, but it was an ectopic pregnancy. After a tubal pregnancy, you have to wait several months before trying to have another baby. The doctor wouldn't put me back on Clomid until my blood pressure was regulated.

I was determined to get my baby with or without his help. So, I started praying and drinking the tea faithfully in February, and by the end of March, I started to suspect I was pregnant, and it was exactly what I expected!

I had my baby girl in November. I recommend it to everyone I know trying to conceive.

-D. R.

Super Cell Food Tea

Superfood #1: Purple Sea Moss—the primary mucus-removing anti-inflammatory ingredient that is highly regarded by Dr. Sebi.

Superfood #2: Bladderwrack—a great choice in the support of a healthy functioning thyroid gland when more iodine is required.

Superfood #3: Burdock root removes toxins from the blood, and it may inhibit some types of cancer.

Superfood #3: Soursop—may help reduce the growth of cancer cells.

I ordered the super cell tea for a friend. She has been dealing with boils under her arms and her "hoohah." She said she can't remember the last time her arms and private area were normal. Y'all, this stuff works.

- C.J.

Everything I have ever ordered from the lab works! It tastes great and works faster than any lupus medication I take! I love the love and time Miss Cotton puts in ALL HER PRODUCTS.

- Whitney

17

Thank You

As I sit here, reflecting on the journey that brought this book to life, I want to take a moment to thank you from the bottom of my heart. Writing this has been deeply personal for me, and knowing that you've taken the time to read it means more than I can express. This isn't just a book—it's a piece of my soul, a collection of lessons I've learned as a child sitting at my grandmother's feet, and with formal training to become a certified Master Herbalist. This is a love letter to the healing power of nature.

I want you to know that everything I've shared here is rooted in my years of study, practice, and personal experience. These aren't just theories or ideas—they're remedies I've used myself, passed on to my family, and watched bring comfort and healing to so many. I truly believe in the power of these plants, and I hope you've felt that belief shine through every page. But here's the thing: this book won't mean much if it just sits on a shelf. I wrote it for you to use.

Try the remedies, brew the teas, and make the salves. Start small if you need to—maybe with a cup of chamomile tea before bed or a lavender sachet tucked into your pillow. It's not about perfection; it's about connection.

When you do, share it. Share what you've learned with your family, your friends, and even your neighbors. These remedies aren't just about healing the body—they're about strengthening the bonds between us. Imagine passing this knowledge down to your children or grandchildren, knowing that they will carry on these traditions long after we're gone. That's the legacy I hope we can build together—a world where natural healing is not just a choice but a way of life.

I know life is busy, and it can feel overwhelming to try something new. Trust me, I've been there. But you don't have to overhaul your entire routine to make a difference. Start by inviting a little piece of nature into your day—a cup of herbal tea, a walk outside, or a small pot of mint growing on your windowsill. Before you know it, these little moments will start to transform the way you live and care for yourself and your loved ones.

Being a Master Herbalist has taught me that healing is as much about intention and love as it is about science. The plants you tend will nourish you in ways you might not expect. They will teach you patience, resilience, and the beauty of slowing down.

So, this is my heartfelt invitation to you: take what you've learned here and make it your own. Use these remedies, adapt them, and share them freely. Let them become part of your family's story, passed down like the most precious heirloom.

Thank you for trusting me to guide you on this journey. Thank you for opening your heart to the wisdom of nature and for being willing to take this first step. I'm honored to have been a part of your life in this way, and I can't wait to see how these traditions grow and thrive in your hands.

With love, gratitude, and all praises to my Creator.

Yolanda Miss Cotton Justice, Certified Master Herbalist

Made in the USA
Monee, IL
04 November 2026

67376095R00085